MW00465505

THEY COULD NOT TALK
AND SO THEY DREW

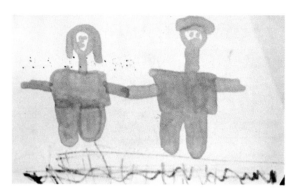
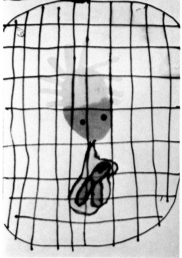
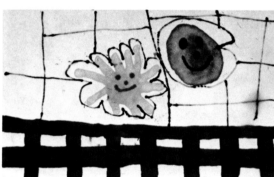
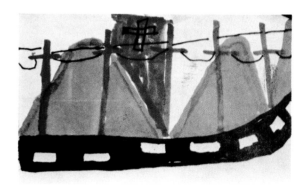

Randy, nine years old, demonstrates advanced levels of cognitive and artistic development in the production of these four watercolor paintings on white paper. His compositions show evidence of identification, introjection, reaction formation and rationalization. In addition, he shows the ability to symbolize, displace, and condense in his image-making, placing him in an equally advanced level of psychosexual development.

THEY COULD NOT TALK AND SO THEY DREW

Children's Styles of Coping and Thinking

By

MYRA F. LEVICK, Ph.D., A.T.R.

Professor and Director of Creative Arts in Therapy Program
Department of Mental Health Sciences
Hahnemann University Graduate School
Philadelphia, Pennsylvania
Charter Member and First President of the
American Art Therapy Association
Editor-in-Chief, The Arts in Psychotherapy: An
International Journal (New York: Ankho International)

Forewords by

Paul J. Fink, M.D.

Professor and Chairman
Department of Psychiatry and Human Behavior
Thomas Jefferson University
Philadelphia, Pennsylvania

and

Zygmunt A. Piotrowski, Ph.D.

Professor, Department of Mental Health Sciences
Hahnemann University
Adjunct Professor, Temple University
Consultant for Research, Medical College of Pennsylvania

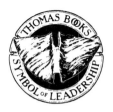

CHARLES C THOMAS • PUBLISHER

Springfield • Illinois • U.S.A.

Published and Distributed Throughout the World by
CHARLES C THOMAS • PUBLISHER
2600 South First Street
Springfield, Illinois, 62717, U.S.A.

This book is protected by copyright. No part of it
may be reproduced in any manner without written
permission from the publisher.

© *1983 by* CHARLES C THOMAS • PUBLISHER
ISBN 0-398-04800-2
Library of Congress Catalog Card Number: 82-19303

With THOMAS BOOKS *careful attention is given to all details of manufacturing and
design. It is the Publisher's desire to present books that are satisfactory as to their physical
qualities and artistic possibilities and appropriate for their particular use.* THOMAS
BOOKS *will be true to those laws of quality that assure a good name and good will.*

Printed in the United States of America
CU-R-1

Library of Congress Cataloging in Publication Data
Levick, Myra F.
    They could not talk and so they drew--children's
styles of coping and thinking.

    Bibliography: p.
    Includes index.
    1. Art therapy.   2. Child psychotherapy.
3. Drawing ability in children.   4. Personality in
children.   5. Cognition in children.   6. Art and
mental illness.   I. title. [DNLM: 1. Art therapy--
In infancy and childhood.   2. Child psychiatry.
WS 350.2 L664t]
RJ505.A7L48   1983   618.92'891656   82-19303
ISBN 0-398-04800-2

This work is dedicated to the three men who more than any other have guided my way: my father, the late Louis Friedman, who taught me to love and to work; the late Morris J. Goldman, M.D., mentor and friend, whose unfaltering belief in art therapy led to the establishment of the first graduate training program in the field and who directed my work; and my husband, Leonard, whose love made it possible for me to grow.

FOREWORD

THIS is an integrative book. Many volumes have been written on Freud and psychosexual development, Piaget and his theories on cognitive development, as well as on the subject of art and its origins, derivatives and meanings. Very few authors have attempted to weave a comprehensive synthesis of all three areas of human mental development and function. Doctor Myra Levick has not only created such a synthesis but has done it in a clear, logical and well-illustrated fashion. The illustrative aspects of this book are both literal and figurative. Using her extraordinary grasp of art therapy, Doctor Levick has allowed us to peer into the drawings of normal children as well as sick children and adults. She has further been able to demonstrate the validity and reliability of her findings regarding the manifestations in art of defense processes in all human beings.

It is sad but true that mental health professionals generally read their own literature and rarely venture out into the intellectual world of their co-workers. The analysts read analytic books and journals for the most part and biologically oriented psychiatrists have a panoply of journals to read which deal primarily with neurobiology and psychopharmacology. Without belaboring the point, there is a cadre of authors and a readership in psychiatry, psychology, social work and the creative arts therapies that all seem to run parallel to one another with little reference to or regard for the important and sometimes crucial discoveries and writings of the other groups.

Doctor Levick started with an idea that germinated through many years as an art therapist, teacher and clinician. She had the conviction that spontaneous artistic production of both normal and abnormal people provided not only a new and different "royal road to the unconscious" but also exposed conflictual and nonconflictual aspects of ego development and function. She and her art therapy colleagues are able to recognize not only the unconscious wishes of the patients but the defensive activities which a person generally uses to cover up, hide from, distort or otherwise keep such wishes out of consciousness. While this has been clear to some of us for many years, the ability to translate artistic material into an understanding of what goes on in the patient's mind is still viewed by many as the unreliable perspicacity of a few talented "sensitive" people with no scientific validity.

Starting with a full appreciation that childhood development may account for adult psychopathology, Doctor Levick still felt a need to integrate the autonomous functions of the ego, the development of cognition with all of its impact on normal and abnormal behavior as well as the special and unique aspects of artistic expression into a single, unified theory. This is an enormous undertaking, and this book, the result of years of observation and study, succeeds in pulling together these three unique and quite different aspects of human endeavor into an approach to the examination and understanding of development and expression.

This book may be viewed from a number of perspectives and hopefully will appeal to a wide readership. First of all, it is a review of three literatures: psychosexual development, Piagetian theory and the nature of artistic production. Secondly, it is a beautiful demonstration of the artistic representation of classical defense mechanisms in the drawings of normal children. Third, it is an overview of pathology in drawings and the presence of pathological defenses consistent with the patient's diagnosis as well as the three interwoven threads that the author has described theoretically earlier in the book. The final way in which this volume may be viewed is as a textbook for art therapists, complete with a firm theoretical framework and charts and tables which guide a budding art therapist to a deeper and clearer understanding and sense of confidence about what they do and their findings both diagnostically and therapeutically.

Using Greenspan primarily as the most recent psychoanalytic developmentalist, Rosen as a clear expositor of Piaget, and Arnheim who has explored the symbolic process, visual imagery and their relationship to art, the first section of the book tries to show how these concepts fit together and how the whole is more meaningful than the sum of the parts. Analysts clearly feel that resistance is a dynamic activity. How then can resistance be presented in a static picture? How can the supposed secondary process, with all of its cognitive elements, present the focus and dynamisms of a primary process activity? How can we see both the unconscious infantile elements and the defenses and resistances inherent in the mental struggle and conflict in the picture that a child or adult presents to us? Doctor Levick attempts to take the three languages used by writers from these three disparate areas and unify them. Careful selection of key authors has made this an eminently readable and useful endeavor. We are introduced to Dabrowski and his hierarchy of values as a bridge between Freud and Piaget. The differences between Dabrowski and Piaget are also carefully explained in order to use both ideas in a better understanding of the creative process and the value of art as a language. We are taken through a series of theoretical discussions, including Greenspan, Noy, Koppitz and DiLeo, in which the author tries to integrate the development of art and drawing with both emotional and cognitive aspects of development.

The clinical sections of this book will help all mental health professionals understand what art therapy is and how it works. Here the seminal work of Anna Freud, *The Ego and the Mechanisms of Defense*, is the foundation upon which this part of the book is built. Age by age and stage by stage, we are guided through an array of pictures which demonstrate the nature of defenses as they appear in both the normal and abnormal. It is like having an expert guide us through a museum. Suddenly, the pictures take on meaning, symbolic and real, and the excitement of the individualized "Rorschach" inherent in art becomes alive. However, this is not just another clinical correlation exercise but an effort to categorize defenses and transform an esoteric specialized area of therapeutic endeavor into a widely applicable activity that is useful to all workers in the field.

This book breaks new ground and catapults art therapy into a new level of theoretical importance within all of psychology. Doctor Levick, long a leader in the field and a staunch supporter of art therapy as a unique subfield of therapeutics intimately related to psychiatry and psychology, has moved into a new position. Through this book she becomes an ambassador of integration and a spokesperson for the development of a common language of human development with a special emphasis on art as a medium of intellectual exchange.

Paul J. Fink

FOREWORD

THIS book expounds two very important and complex scientific problems: (1) which are the mental and behavioral processes
essential to interpersonal relationships that are revealed by a child's
free drawings — drawings of lines, all sorts of figures, particularly
human — and (2) how can the child's developmental level be ascer-
tained by an analysis of his drawings. Doctor Levick advances the
solution of the problem of the relation between the visual-motor imagery which created the drawings and the child's psychosocial
behavior, conscious and unconscious, overt and latent. Her work
has both practical and theoretical significance. During the first years
of life, non-verbal communication is by far more meaningful than
the limited verbal speech of early childhood. The non-verbal, early
childhood is the period of the most intense growth and maturation,
and the engrams of the strongest early childhood experiences are
likely to exert a lifelong, albeit unconscious, influence. This ac-
counts for the stability and power of imagery. The hands and the
eyes play a dominant role in learning about the world and adapting
to it. Hands and eyes also play a decisive role in executing drawings,
in giving external form to the non-verbal imaginary conceptions of
the brain which is the source of the child's more or less organized
conscious and unconscious adaptive activities and intentions.
Throughout our entire life the brain never sleeps. Thus the imagery
is kept alive also in adulthood and keeps changing ceaselessly with
changing, expanding and new experiences that matter to us.

Of great interest and value is Doctor Levick's establishing a connection between the development of Piaget's cognitive mechanisms
and Freud's libidinal levels. Instead of viewing the two schemes as
incompatible and competitive, she views them as compatible and
complementary. After all, nothing is ever done without an affective
impulse even when the affect is ever so feeble because the action does
not matter very much to us. Affects signify a readiness to act. At the
same time, we must mobilize our knowledge pertinent to a suc-

cessful performing of the intended action. We must know the reality conditions that would facilitate or obstruct the carrying out of the desired activity. As affects and cognition are inseparable and necessary subjective processes of living, Freud's psychodynamic scheme of the child's development and Piaget's scheme of the development of the child's cognitive functions supplement one another. This synthesis gives us a fuller and more meaningful conception of the process of personality maturation in childhood. Doctor Levick has demonstrated the chronological correspondence between Freud's and Piaget's stages in the process of development. These stages are illustrated by actual clinical cases and clinical material. The emphasis is on specific graphic elements and their connection with affective and thinking symptoms.

There is also a discussion of drawings produced by schizophrenics — adolescents as well as adults. These are qualitatively different from children's drawings. It seems more difficult to change deliberately and diagnose elements of graphic productions than words or overt body movements. Drawings of human figures easily reveal the internal changes contingent upon the schizophrenic disease process. Sometimes a glance at a drawing reveals the psychosis when other evidence is ambiguous. In these cases, the drawings exhibit conspicuously the condition of the patient's sense of reality, his rigidity, withdrawal, and bizarreness of emotions. Attitudes toward sex play a prominent role in the preoccupations of schizophrenics. Separate drawings of a man and a woman made by early or mild cases frequently differ strikingly, revealing an inner mental state differing noticeably from the overt, manifest mental state. This difference is prognostically as well as therapeutically important. The traits that make the figure of the same sex (as that of the patient) differ from the other-sex figure are assented and expressed in manifest behavior, with greater ease and frequency than are those traits which make the other-sex figure differ from the same-sex figure. Individuals habitually try to control or inhibit the overt manifestation of those traits which they assign exclusively to their other-sex figures in spontaneous free drawings; or they disclose them in their behavior in special situations of increased tension, such as great anxiety, unexpected temptation or irritating provocation. Graphic productions of children and adults betray a greater influence of genuine affects and intentions than do their more disciplined public speaking and motor behavior.

This volume contains a constructive survey of pertinent literature, case samples and a list of definitions of Piaget's concepts referring to cognitive growth. Aside of advancing the psychological interpretation of children's free drawings, it offers a unique correlation of Freud's and Piaget's stages of the child's maturation. It is an instructive and original work.

Zygmunt A. Piotrowski

PREFACE

THIS work represents the culmination of my educational and professional experience as a clinical art psychotherapist and educator in the field of creative arts in therapy. While emanating from a specific area of psychoanalytic theory — defense mechanisms of the ego — the relationship between cognitive and psychosexual development and the relationship between imagery and thinking and learning are explored.

The literature on art therapy, defense mechanisms of the ego, Piagetian theory and artistic development relevant to the scope of this work is reviewed. A synthesis of this material through the text and illustrations of spontaneous and directed drawings by normal children aged two to ten years follow. This age group was selected because the literature strongly suggests that by around age ten most children have acquired a repertoire of defense mechanisms that enable them to make the transition through adolescence to adulthood. Numerous examples of drawings produced by emotionally disturbed children and adults are also presented along with a text describing the developmental manifestation of maladaptive defense mechanisms of the ego and their relationship to cognitive, psychosexual, and artistic development as they are manifested in the same drawing.

In retrospect, I can see how the beginning of the wish to pursue this endeavor took hold in the earliest years of my training in art therapy, grew stronger as I began to teach, and slowly evolved like the pieces of a jigsaw puzzle coming together.

Once the format, described above, was clearly envisioned and all the references and illustrations were at hand, there remained only the task of defining my criteria for identifying defense mechanisms in drawings on a hierarchical scale. Accomplishing this, I soon learned the puzzle was larger than I had anticipated. It became apparent that to describe my assumptions and illustrate them through drawings and tables was not enough.

xv

Originally, there was no intent to include any statistical analysis of my thesis. I believed in proposing a theory; it remained for others to test it. The challenge to incorporate some measure of reliability and validity in this work came from several directions, including my own awareness that documentations of theoretical constructs in art therapy and even psychiatry lag far behind other areas of psychology. So, in spite of my initial resistance and even trepidation and with the support of those who are acknowledged later, two studies were subsequently implemented.

The first, a reliability study, was conducted, and I thank Ronald E. Hays and Susan Kaye-Huntington, both former students and now colleagues, for consenting to serve as blind raters for a random distribution of the illustrations. The second study examined the validity of my criteria for identifying defense mechanisms in drawings, and I thank the four psychotherapists who participated in this study but must remain anonymous to preserve the confidentiality of their patients.

The reliability study demonstrated significantly high interrater reliability and there was a high percentage of agreement and no significant difference between the number of defenses identified by the four psychotherapists and myself. The tables showing these results and a discussion of their implications appear in the Appendices.

As the pieces begin to fall into place and complete the "picture," they demonstrate that defense mechanisms and intelligence (a function of the conflict-free sphere of the ego), as manifested in spontaneous or directed drawings of children and adults, provide significant information regarding an individual's capacity for adaptation to reality.

Members of education and mental health disciplines, other than art therapists, can use graphic productions to discern whether or not a child or an adult has age-appropriate capabilities. Thus, the knowledgeable evaluation of spontaneous and even directed drawings is provided with a sensitive, serviceable schema.

Myra F. Levick

INTRODUCTION

THE facts and fantasies, data vis-à-vis spontaneous drawings, old concepts and new constructs to be presented in these chapters reflect a personal experience over two decades in training and as clinical art-psychotherapist and educator in the field of the creative arts in therapy. This process can be likened to the developmental stages of cognitive and emotional growth described in what have been traditionally two separate bodies of literature. Numerous psychologists and psychoanalysts have historically deplored the schism between Piagetian and psychoanalytic theory and many have put forth constructs connecting the two schools of thought. Some of these will be cited.

The following chapters are not only the culmination of the educational and professional experiences noted but also a synthesis of these experiences emanating from a specific area of psychoanalytic theory: defense mechanisms of the ego. To clarify how this came about and subsequently to be the focus of this work, I shall describe briefly the course of my own development.

Because of what I now consider a most fortunate set of circumstances in 1963, I had the opportunity to utilize my talent and training as a painter in a twenty-nine bed inpatient unit for adults suffering from moderate neurosis to severe psychosis. At the same time, I was required to attend intensive in-service training in psychoanalytic theory. My job title was "art therapist" and one of my first tasks was to learn what that implied. Fortunately, there was some literature not too many years before in this field by Margaret Naumburg, Edith Kramer, Elinor Ulman and Ernst Harms.

Their major contributions, and those that followed, will be reviewed in an overview of art therapy. At that time, their writings (which consisted primarily of their individual philosophies and case material), coupled with the training I was receiving, became the basis for my own development as an art therapist. I gravitated toward the dynamically oriented approach described by Ms. Naumburg and found it most helpful in integrating theory and practice. The focus was on psychopathology, manifestations of mental disorders and adaptive and maladaptive ego-defense mechanisms in the drawings of patients referred for art therapy. The frame of reference for defining these elements in graphic images was the psychoanalytic theory of developmental stages (i.e. oral, anal and Oedipal stages). Examples of these will be given. While strengths and weaknesses of ego function and intellectual capacity were considered, they were not paramount in making diagnoses or interpretations in the process of therapy. Exposure to organicity (i.e. brain damage) was limited and only seen occasionally in the repetitive drawings of senile geriatric patients. Normal development was identified by its absence in the population I worked with. This deficiency became glaringly apparent during graduate work in educational psychology. Exposure to learning theory and behavioral psychology was both stimulating and frustrating. There was little in the literature at that time (1965) that constructively integrated the separate schools of thought.

In 1967, I became responsible for developing a program to train art therapists in the graduate school that was part of Hahnemann Medical College and Hospital. In spite of my educational experience with other theories mentioned above, I was convinced (and still am) that an understanding of psychoanalytic theory was essential in training art therapists to work with a variety of populations living with some form of mental dysfunction. Although introduction to the numerous psychological theories was incorporated in the original curriculum (and these theories continue to be redefined and integrated), the core of the psychology courses was and is psychoanalytic theory. My own particular interest and expertise evolved around ego mechanisms of defense: how they reflected adaptive and maladaptive behavior patterns, how they reflected developmental stages in terms of areas of unresolved conflict leading to fixations in developmental stages and, specifically, how these elements are manifested in drawings of children and adults in a therapeutic milieu.

Subsequently, several incidents occurred which impressed me with the need to learn much more about normal cognitive and emotional development and their relationship to each other, and how mechanisms of defense reflected these on a continuum. The latter is indeed only one aspect of multiple ego functions but in my view plays a significant role in personality development. Knowledge of defense mechanisms of the ego and how individuals utilize them provides inferences about total personality development, particularly when identified within the gestalt of graphic images produced by normal and abnormal populations.

Stated briefly, among incidents that led to further learning was one at a national conference of the American Society for the Psychopathology of Expression, where I was compelled to recognize the implications of the interaction of cognitive and emotional systems in a presentation by Leslie Osborne, M.D. He described his experiences during a term as a state mental health director and the shocking discovery that some inmates of an institution for the mentally retarded had average and above-average intellectual capacities even though their scores on intelligence tests were between forty-five and sixty-five. His initial suspicions were based on observations of their ability to appropriately draw objects in their environment and to make complex constructions from tiny pieces of Leggo® (a sophisticated construction toy). His concerns were well documented in subsequent programs and evaluations implemented at that institution. His results forced our faculty to take a hard look at the whole issue along developmental lines and to identify manifestations of cognitive skills and emotional states in drawings produced by normal and abnormal populations in order to learn more about the relationship and interaction of these two domains. Another incident involved a member of our hospital psychiatric staff who was serving on the thesis committee for one of our students. Throughout the years, a number of our students hypothesized that certain defenses are specific to certain mental disorders and, therefore, they focused their research on testing this hypothesis through manifestations of the defenses in the drawings of patients with specific diagnoses. While a number of art therapists have written case studies based on one or more defense mechanisms identified in the drawings of these patients, our psychiatrist expressed his frustration over the fact that there was no comprehensive text addressing this subject and suggested I write one since I was teaching in the field. Although willing to attempt such a project, I had a gnawing notion that this had to be reviewed and reported in conjunction with cognitive development. More graduate work in child development was essential, and this, joined with my research in the relationship between cognitive and psychosexual development, and the relationship between imagery and thinking and learning, filled in some of the gaps sufficiently to allow for the writing of this book.

The need to integrate psychoanalytic and Piagetian developmental psychology has produced some noteworthy literature. The intent of this work is not to present a comprehensive review of the literature pertaining to the integration of these two theories. Rather, the literature that is specifically relevant to this material will be noted in the related context. A most excellent theoretical construct integrating these two schools was authored by Greenspan (1979). His work, including some of the review of the literature, will be referred to more frequently than any other in this area. The works of Anna Freud (1936, 1965, 1966) are the basis for the theoretical orientation presented here.

To focus on one aspect of ego function is not without its problems.

> If, as in 1936, it was sufficient to enumerate and illustrate ego mechanisms, to inquire into their chronology, and to assess the role of the defense organization as a whole for the maintenance of health or illness, this can no longer be done today without relating the ego's defensive achievements to its other aspects, i.e., to its primary deficiencies, its apparatuses and functions, its autonomy, etc. (A. Freud, 1966).

However, there is some support for this limited approach. Hartman (1939) and Greenspan (1979) point out the need for a hierarchical developmental model of ego substructures that is concerned with adaptation and reality. Hartman states that the choice of defense mechanisms results from both constitutional determinants and the maturation of the conflict-free sphere of the ego. It is the goal of our presentation to demonstrate that defense mechanisms and intelligence (a function of the conflict-free sphere of the ego), as manifested in spontaneous or directed drawings of children and adults, provide significant information regarding an individual's capacity for adaptation to reality. Ego strengths and ego weaknesses cannot be defined without consideration of those ego functions that serve as a base for intelligent behavior and behaviors emanating from will and action (Greenspan, 1979). Greenspan also points out that from his clinical experience it is apparent that "content of children's play, fantasy and imitation is often related to emotional issues." Therefore, he believes expression cannot be fully understood from a cognitive viewpoint, but those elements related to the influence of drives and object relations must be considered. Rappaport (1954) maintains that repression, ideational representation, and (less directly) affect discharge result in internalization of reality and its representation in the psychic apparatus. He also contends that "every mechanism we observe corresponds to such a counter-cathectic energy distribution. These defensive apparatuses come to our attention in the form of motivations of behavior, such as denial, avoidance, altruism, honesty, etc." (p. 255).

Finally, mention must be made of an ever-present concept — resistance. Moore and Fine (1968) define this term as

> a phenomenon encountered in the course of psychoanalytic treatment. This psychic equilibrium of a person rests on the balance of inner psychic forces, and the disturbance of the equilibrium causes anxiety. People tend, therefore, to oppose automatically anything that disturbs the inner balance, regardless of the fact that they may know that the interference with the established balance might be to their long-term advantage . . . During the psychoanalytic treatment the patient is encouraged to talk about activities going on in his mind. As he does so . . . , he becomes increasingly aware of the prohibitive-defense part of his mind as well as wishes and urges which are held in check by the prohibitions . . . (p. 87).

It seems, therefore, that resistance is at the core of adaptive and maladaptive developmental behaviors. It follows that insofar as this orientation to art therapy is analogous to psychoanalytic theory and practice (i.e. psychosexual development, dream interpretation and free association), understanding and identifying defense mechanisms and their relationship to cognitive skills from a developmental perspective in drawings can be particularly useful to not only psychoanalysts and art psychotherapists but to psychologists and other clinicians in the field of mental health. In addition, there is a cadre of educators confronted with the national mandate that all children have a right to education regardless of handicap (P.L. 94-142), who may also benefit from this guide to assessing adaptation to reality in children's drawings.

The following chapters will present an overview of art therapy in this country, a review of the literature on defense mechanisms relevant to this work, aspects of the relationship between cognitive and psychosexual development as it pertains to drawings and, lastly, examples of these elements in the drawings of normal children two to ten years of age and in the drawings of mentally dysfunctioning children and adults.

ACKNOWLEDGMENTS

I WANT to thank Doctor Samuel Snyder, formerly in Department of Education and Child Development, Bryn Mawr College, to whom I first presented the idea for this work. He thought it was very worthwhile and encouraged its development. I am grateful to Janet Hoopes, Ph.D., Chairperson, Department of Education and Child Development, Bryn Mawr College, who gave generously of her time and expertise in clinical assessment and supported my efforts to suggest new directions in this area. Without the support and encouragement of Israel Zwerling, M.D., Ph.D., chairperson of the Department of Mental Health Sciences at Hahnemann Medical College and Hospital, and the patience and consideration of my staff, Dianne Dulicai, Cynthia Briggs, Ron Hays and our secretary, Doris Klayman, I could not have had the time necessary to prepare for and complete this manuscript.

It was a privilege to have had the opportunity to consult with Herman Belmont, M.D., deputy chairman of Child Psychiatry, Hahnemann Medical College and Hospital. His knowledge of child development and psychoanalytic theory is renowned, and his comments and thoughts forced me to write with greater clarity.

I want to express my warm gratitude to Paul J. Fink, M.D., chairman of the Department of Psychiatry and Human Behavior, Thomas Jefferson University, who also read this manuscript as it evolved. His years of teaching and writing in the area of art therapy and his professional and personal interest in this effort made him a sensitive and invaluable critic.

Two special friends, Paul Cutler, M.D., physician and author, and Harry Cohen, M.D., psychoanalyst, voluntarily offered to read the first draft. Their interest and support at that initial phase spurred me on.

There were many colleagues, relatives and friends who collected their children's drawings and sent them to me who must remain anonymous to preserve confidentiality. A number of nursery school directors and teachers who either sent me drawings or allowed me to observe and work with their students must also remain anonymous for the same reason. Their cooperation and consideration is gratefully appreciated; their contributions enrich this presentation. A special thanks to my daughter, Karen, who spent many summer weeks cataloguing these pictures.

I was fortunate to have two excellent typists, Nicoletta Berd and Sally Sylk, whose interest in the subject matter made our working arrangements very special and productive. Their work was made easier by the excellent editing by my good friend Sylvia Halpern, and the proofreading was completed by another good friend, Helene Cutler.

Thanks must also be given here to the numbers of students I have taught over the years who have prodded me to put this method of assessment down on paper. Their belief in its usefulness had significant influence on this undertaking. On behalf of these students and myself, I want to take this occasion to thank V. Michael Vaccaro, M.D. His knowledge of psychiatry coupled with a remarkable sensitivity to the graphic images produced by psychotic patients led to our joint effort in formulating the original course in art therapy theory taught in the program at Hahnemann Medical College and Hospital. Our continued striving to communicate verbally that which seemed so clear on the non-verbal level is at the root of this endeavor.

Lastly, I want to thank my family, who acknowledged my priorities often before their own, and especially my grandsons, Brent and Keith, who continue to draw pictures for me.

CONTENTS

Page

Foreword by Paul J. Fink..................................... vii

Foreword by Zygmunt A. Piotrowski........................... xi

Preface xv

Introduction xvii

Chapter

1. ART THERAPY: AN OVERVIEW............................. 3
   Definition.. 3
   History.. 4
   Theory.. 8
   Methodology 10
   Applications... 11
   Summary.. 14

2. DEFENSE MECHANISMS OF THE EGO: A DEVELOPMENTAL
   PERSPECTIVE.. 16
   Historical Overview..................................... 16
   Chronological Development of Defenses.................... 20
   Summary.. 28

3. PSYCHOSEXUAL AND COGNITIVE DEVELOPMENT: THEIR
   RELATIONSHIP TO DEVELOPMENTAL SEQUENCES IN CHILDREN'S
   DRAWINGS: A THEORETICAL OVERVIEW 30
   Piagetian Theory.. 31
   Piagetian and Psychoanalytic Theories: A View Towards
      Integration 36
   Developmental Sequences in Children's Drawings: Emotional
      and Cognitive Factors................................. 44
   Relationship Between Cognitive Development and Artistic Skill. 53
   Development of Language and Relationship to Visual Imagery.. 57
   Summary.. 59

Chapter *Page*

4. MANIFESTATIONS OF DEFENSE MECHANISMS IN CHILDREN'S
   DRAWINGS: RELATIONSHIP TO PSYCHOSEXUAL AND COGNITIVE
   DEVELOPMENTAL ASPECTS IN DRAWINGS 63
     Three and Four Years of Age............................. 66
     Five to Seven Years of Age.............................. 75
     Seven to Eleven Years of Age........................... 94
     Summary 109
5. MANIFESTATIONS OF DEFENSE MECHANISMS IN THE DRAWINGS
   OF DISTURBED CHILDREN AND YOUNG ADULTS 133
6. CONCLUSION 161

   Appendix 171
   Glossary of Piagetian Terms.............................. 191
   Bibliography 197
   Index 201

TABLES

Table   *Page*

1 Correlation of Developmental Lines of Cognitive, Artistic, Psychosexual Sequences and Defense Mechanisms
of the Ego Appropriate for Those Periods of
Development 61

2 Definitions and Criteria for Identifying Defenses Mani-
fested in Graphic Productions 129

3 Defense Mechanisms of the Ego Identified in a Random
Sample of Drawings by Two Blind Raters and Correlated
with Those Identified by the Author in Those Same
Drawings 172

4 Number of Defense Mechanisms Identified by Author
and Two Raters; Number Raters Were in Agreement
with Author; Number They Omitted; Number
They Added 178

5 Raters' Responses Correlated with Author and Each
Other Using Pearson Product Moment Statistical
Test 181

6 Intraclass r (based on a 1-way ANOVA) k = 3; r = 46
(No. of Phenomena Examined by All Three Raters) 182

7 Comparison of Defenses Identified in Drawings by
Author (A) and Defenses Identified in Behavior by
Psychologist/Psychiatrist (P) 184

8 Number and Percent of Agreement between A and P on
Total Possible Number of Defense Mechanisms of
the Ego (DEF) 186

9 Number and Percent Agreement of A with 8 of Defenses
Present and Defenses Absent 187

10 A & P Responses of # Absent Correlated Using Pearson
Product Moment Statistical Test 188

11 Chi Square Contingency Table
Assumption: Presence and Absence of each Defense was
Independent Variable 189

THEY COULD NOT TALK
AND SO THEY DREW

Chapter One

ART THERAPY: AN OVERVIEW*

Definition

A RT therapy as a discipline has grown rapidly during the last twenty years and its definition has gone through many changes. "Since the time of the caveman, men have created configurations which serve as equivalents for life processes" (1958, p. 7). Kramer also describes art as a means of widening the scope of human experience by providing a way to express these experiences through various art media. She further states, "The art therapist assists in an act of integration and synthesis" (p. 21). Fink, Levick and Goldman define art therapy as that discipline which combines elements of psychotherapy with untapped sources of creativity and expression in the patient (1967, p. 2). Levick (1967) maintains that art therapy should be considered as a "prescribed substitution of creative activity to replace neurotic symptoms and to strengthen defenses successfully by the patient before illness becomes acute, and establish a prescribed relationship with the therapist" (p. 158). This relationship is in accord with the treatment goals for the patient.

With the development of training in the field of art therapy, the need for further clarification became evident. In an early pamphlet of the American Art Therapy Association (established in 1969), an attempt was made to describe the goal of art therapy as "help for the individual child or adult to find a more compatible relationship between his inner and outer worlds."

The current definition given by the American Art Therapy Association is:

Art therapy provides the opportunity for nonverbal expression and communication. Within the field there are two major approaches. The use of art as therapy implies that the creative process can be a means both of reconciling emotional conflicts and of fostering self-awareness and personal growth. When using art as a vehicle for psychotherapy, both the

*Levick, M.F. Art therapy: an overview. In Corsini, R. (Ed.): *Handbook of Innovative Psychotherapies* (New York: John Wiley & Sons, 1981, pp. 51-58). Reprinted by permission of John Wiley & Sons, Inc.

3

product and the associative references may be used in an effort to help the individual find a more compatible relationship between his inner and outer worlds.

Art therapy like art education may teach technique and media skills. When art is used as therapy the instruction provides a vehicle for self-expression, communication and growth. Less product oriented, the art therapist is more concerned with the individual's inner experience. Process, form, content, and/or associations become important for what each reflects about personality development, personality traits and the unconscious.

As can be noted from the above, definitions have gone from the specific to the more general interpretation of art therapy. Although the current definition seems to suffice in most areas, the field continues to grow and develop not one but several approaches to the process of art therapy. Consequently, this may eventually demand several specific definitions rather than a single encompassing one.

History

The late Ernst Harms, founder and former editor of the *International Journal of Art Psychotherapy*, traced the healing effects of the arts (in this case, music) back to biblical sources which describe how David tried to cure King Saul's depression by playing the harp (Harms, 1976). Kraeplin (1912) and Bleuler (1918) also suggested that drawings by patients be considered in making diagnoses. Printzhorn's book, published in 1922, spurred outstanding psychopathologists to use the art expressions of patients to diagnose their pathological conditions. Hammer (1958) states, "From these causal diagnostic beginnings, a great number of systematic diagnostic methods have been developed which today we call tests; and the method has been designed as a projective technique (in Harms, 1976)."

In 1925, Nolan C. Lewis began to use free painting with adult neurotics. Stern (1952) described free painting in psychoanalysis with adult neurotics and stated that one of the reasons that this modality had not been generally adopted might have been in part a lack of understanding in the use of the technique.

"Art therapy as a profession was first defined in America in the writings of Margaret Naumburg" (Levick, 1973, p. 237). Naumburg dates her awareness of the relationship between children's drawings and psychotherapy to her early years of experience as director and art teacher of the Walden School, which she founded in 1915. She became convinced that the free art expression of children represented a symbolic form of speech that was basic to all education. As the years passed, she concluded that this "form of spontaneous art expression was also basic to psychotherapeutic treatment" (Naumburg, 1947, 1966, p. 30).

Under the direction of Doctor Nolan C. Lewis, she initiated an experimental research program in the use of spontaneous art in therapy with behavior-problem children at the New York State Psychiatric Unit. The results of the study were first published in 1947. In 1958, graduate courses in the principles and methods of her concept of dynamically oriented art therapy were instituted at New York University in New York City. Her prolific writings, lectures, and seminars throughout the country spearheaded growing interest in the field and stimulated mental health professionals and educators to question and explore the possibilities of a broader conceptual framework in the application of art as a diagnostic and therapeutic tool.

Subsequent art therapists, some trained by Naumburg, added significant impetus to the development of this modality and should be mentioned briefly. Elinor Ulman early on defined her profession as an art teacher and took some training in art education through lectures and seminars at the Washington School of Psychiatry and a series of lectures on art therapy by Naumburg. In the early 1950s she took a position in a psychiatric clinic. She later worked at the District of Columbia General Hospital where Doctor Bernard Levy, chief psychologist, taught her the principles of diagnosis (Ulman, 1966). In 1961, she published the first issue of the *Bulletin of Art Therapy*, which has continued to be a major publication in the field.

Ben Ploger has been both an art teacher and art therapist. He began teaching art in Houston, Texas in 1935. He studied music, was a lay minister and was professor and chairman of the Department of Fine Arts at Delgado College in New Orleans. In the early 1960s he was persuaded by a psychiatric nurse to volunteer time to teach art to mentally disturbed nuns cloistered in the religious unit of the De Paul Hospital. He soon began to introduce and implement his own expertise throughout the hospital and was made director of art psychotherapy there in 1966. He was a charter member of the American Art Therapy Association and the first chairman of the

Standards Committee.

In 1950, Edith Kramer initiated and for nine years thereafter conducted an art therapy program at Wiltwyck School for Boys in New York City. Her first book, *Art Therapy in a Children's Community*, was written in 1958. Kramer is widely known as a lecturer and teacher in the field and is currently on the faculty of the graduate program of art therapy at New York University in New York City.

During the Second World War, Don Jones, a conscientious objector, volunteered for duty at Marlboro State Hospital in New Jersey. In a letter, he stated, "Having had an art background before, I immediately became intrigued by the many graphic productions and projections of patients which literally covered the walls of some rooms and of passageways between different buildings." In 1950, while teaching painting classes at Kansas University, he met a number of psychiatrists and social workers from the Menninger Clinic who were his students. He was introduced to Doctor Karl Menninger and shared with him a manuscript and paintings reflecting his wartime experience. This resulted in his being employed as an art therapist at the Menninger Foundation and was the beginning of the art therapy program there. Jones stayed on until 1966. Since then he has been director of the Adjunctive Therapy Department at Harding Hospital in Worthington, Ohio. He is also a past president of the American Art Therapy Association.

In 1967, the late Doctor Morris Goldman became director of the Hahnemann Community Mental Health Center in Philadelphia, and, within a few months, he and Doctor Paul Fink, then director of education and training of the Department of Psychiatry at Hahnemann Medical College and Hospital, proposed the first graduate training program in art therapy in the world, leading to a master's degree at that institution. It is this program that was discussed in the Introduction.

In 1968, Hahnemann Medical College and Hospital hosted a lecture series in art therapy for practicing art therapists throughout the country. An *ad hoc* committee was elected to develop guidelines for the organization of a national art therapy association. The committee members were Elinor Ulman, Don Jones, Felice Cohen (a well-known art therapist at Texas Research Institute in Houston, Texas), Robert Ault (art therapist at the Menninger Foundation, who had been trained by Don Jones and who replaced Jones when he left Menninger), and myself. In 1969, the American Art Therapy Association was officially launched in Louisville, Kentucky.

The art therapists mentioned here reflect only a small number of the highly competent men and women who were ultimately responsible for establishing art therapy as a profession in America and abroad.

The American Art Therapy Association has designated professional entry into the field at the master's or graduate level training in institute or clinical programs. Graduate training must include didactic and practicum experience, but the emphasis may vary depending on the facility in which the student is trained. A master's degree from an accredited academic institution or a certificate of completion from an accredited institute or clinical program is supported by the American Art Therapy Association as professional qualification for entry into the field. Accredited undergraduate programs that provide basic areas of fine arts and the behavioral sciences in preparation for graduate training are also supported by the American Art Therapy Association. These two areas are prerequisites for specialized art therapy training in the history, theory, and practice of art therapy.

The association has also developed specific standards for registration, and art therapists who have met these standards receive a certificate of registration by the AATA and may use the initials ATR after their names. There are now approximately 2,000 members of the association.

In 1974, Gantt and Strauss prepared a bibliography through a grant from the National Institute of Mental Health. It is a comprehensive, annotated bibliography of literature in the field of art therapy from 1940 to 1973. There are two major publications: (1) *The American Journal of Art Therapy* (previously, *Journal of Art Therapy*) [Editor, Elinor Ulman, Washington, D.C.]; and (2) *The Arts in Psychotherapy: An International Journal* [Editors-in-Chief, Myra F. Levick and Edith Wallace; Publisher, ANKHO International, Inc., New York].

Art therapists work in public and private institutions treating a variety of mental disorders and in public schools and private schools for the learning-disabled child and mentally and physically handicapped child and adult. More recently, art therapy has been employed with terminally ill and physically disabled persons. Art therapy is practiced with individuals, groups, and/or families.

Theory

Not all practicing art therapists view man's behavior as a product of unconscious thoughts and feelings. Current training in the field embraces many orientations; therefore it follows that the philosophy of art therapists coming from theoretical frameworks, such as behavioral modification, Gestalt, client-centered, humanistic, etc., would be different from that originally put forth by Ms. Naumburg: "Most drawings of the emotionally disordered express problems involving certain polarities, e.g., life–death, male–female, father–mother, love–hate, activity versus passivity, space, rhythm, color, some being specialized and others being generalized in composition" (Naumburg, 1947, p. v).

The psychoanalytic approach to ego mechanisms of defense is the basis for treatment methods in art therapy (Naumburg, 1966). Naumburg maintains that spontaneous art expression releases unconscious material and that the transference relation between patient and therapist plays an important role in the therapeutic process. Ulman (1961) holds that the encouragement of free association in pictures clearly allies dynamic art therapy with psychoanalytic therapy.

More recent proponents of Naumburg's original premise believe that the patient's artistic productions, like the dream brought to the analyst, cannot be interpreted without the patient's associations. Condensation, displacement, symbolism, secondary elaboration, components of dreams and graphic productions, plus the patient's associations, provide more information than is often observable in the clinical setting (Fink, 1967).

In 1958, a second and widely respected theory of art therapy was formulated by Edith Kramer. While recognizing the unconscious as a determinant for man's behavior, she believes that the very act of creating is healing; that the *art* in therapy provides a means of widening the range of human experience by "creating equivalents for such experiences" (Ulman, 1961, p. 13).

Kramer places great emphasis on the process of sublimation, and high value on the arts in the treatment process of the mentally ill. She clearly identifies her role with patients as different from that of the art teacher, in that the process takes precedence over the product. At Wiltwyck School, Kramer was "at once artist, therapist and teacher" (Ulman, 1961, p. 12).

Art therapists who have adopted the Naumburg orientation are viewed as psychotherapists by the followers of Kramer; art therapists who, like Kramer, place emphasis on the healing quality of the creative process are viewed as art teachers (Ulman, 1961). The current literature which primarily consists of case studies reflects a wide variety of theoretical concepts somewhere between Naumburg and Kramer. Many of these theoretical formulations and methodologies have evolved as the result of the many different graduate training programs established throughout this country in the past eight years. As briefly suggested above, there were a number of pioneers in the field who developed their own unique art therapy theories based on years of experience rather than a single theoretical frame of reference.

For those dynamically oriented art therapists, the goal is to allow the transference relationship to develop so that through the patients' associations to their spontaneous drawings insights into conflictual areas of the psyche may be uncovered. In the process of making verbal what was nonverbal, conscious what was unconscious, the art psychotherapist makes connections and clarifications in an effort to help the patient interpret his/her own symbolic images.

In placing emphasis on the healing aspect of the creative process, the goal of art therapy is to provide a means, according to Kramer, "wherein experiences can be chosen, varied, repeated at will" (Ulman, 1961, p. 13). It also provides an opportunity to re-experience conflict and then to resolve and to integrate the resolution.

As previously noted, there are no longer just two accepted divergent viewpoints, but many viable frames of reference that provide a basis for establishing treatment goals. Although I was trained in a psychoanalytically oriented milieu, years of experience as a therapist and educator have demonstrated that the most valid goal is that which is consistent with the needs of the patient/client regardless of theoretical orientation. Whatever the viewpoint is, the most valid goals would be as follows: "(1) provide a means for strengthening the ego; (2) provide a cathartic experience; (3) provide a means to uncover anger; (4) offer an avenue to reduce guilt; (5) facilitate a task to develop impulse control; (6) introduce an experience to help develop the ability to integrate and relate; and (7) help patients/ clients use art as a new outlet during an incapacitating illness" (Levick, 1967).

Methodology

The clinical application of art therapy encompasses the hospitalized child and adult, psychotic and neurotic populations voluntarily seeking some form of psychiatric intervention or treatment, prison populations, mentally retarded populations, learning-disabled children, troubled couples and families and, more recently, those individuals manifesting emotional problems resulting from physical illnesses such as chronic kidney disease, cancer, hemophilia, asthma, diabetes, and neurological diseases.

Art therapy sessions may be conducted on a one-to-one basis in small or large groups and with families. They may be held in the art therapist's office, the classroom, the dining room of an inpatient unit, or the basement of a general hospital. This is contingent on the needs and orientation of the director or administrator of the institution that employs an art therapist and the orientation and style of the art therapist in private practice.

Specific methods and techniques vary for the reasons mentioned above. However, it is generally accepted within the profession that the art therapist must have a sound knowledge of and considerable experience with all art media in order to carry out the varied treatment goals in the art therapy session. For example, finger paint, oil paints, and clay are tactile media that foster the compulsion to smear. If the treatment goal is to provide structure towards helping the patient gain internal controls, these supplies would not be helpful and could be detrimental to the goal. A more productive choice of media might be felt-tipped markers or crayons.

Patients who need to be encouraged to communicate with others, because they cannot do so verbally, often benefit from some form of group-mural activity.

For the child who has become either withdrawn or a behavior problem because of a specific learning disability, the first drawing accepted and valued by the art therapist/teacher may be the first step towards self-acceptance for that child.

For all patients/clients, art therapy — a non-verbal form of communication — provides a way to gain distance from disturbing thoughts and feelings. For the psychotic patient, it often helps to separate fantasy from fact; for the severely neurotic patient, it may help connect feelings and thoughts.

For troubled families, art therapy may dispel family myths and uncover denied scapegoating. Unhealthy alliances can be confronted and changed, and healthy separation of generations and consequent individuation can be reinforced.

Drawings done by chronic, long-term, inarticulate patients often serve as the only means of evaluating prognosis, establishing treatment goals and determining discharge procedures.

The length of therapy varies with the setting in which it is conducted and with the orientation of the therapist. Just as any other form of psychotherapy conducted in a short-term hospital unit, art therapy would be consistent with the treatment goals of the milieu. In a one-to-one situation where the art therapist has a therapeutic contract with the patient, the length of therapy would reflect both the needs of the patient and the therapist's clinical application of his/her particular orientation.

Applications

Art therapy has demonstrated its efficacy with a variety of populations and diagnoses. The most prevalent of these is schizophrenia, probably due to the fact that the schizophrenic patient, suffering an acute episode, is usually in a severe state of regression and "seems compelled to express himself compulsively and continually through any art media" (Levick, 1975, p. 93). Spontaneous drawings and associations are elicited and used to gain a better understanding of areas of conflict. "The art therapist offers the patient clarifications, connections, confrontations, and interpretations depending on the patient's capacity to handle the material being expressed" (Levick, 1975, p. 94).

There is a need for caution in providing oil paints to the older adult schizophrenic patient. This medium may foster regression and thus overwhelm the patient. The following, however, is an example of an exception in which the therapist devised a method that prevented regression for the schizophrenic patient and provided encouragement:

> A man in his early thirties, who had previously demonstrated some artistic
> talent, communicated that he wished to paint in oils. On his own, he ob-
> tained the medium and was later observed in great distress. He had stop-
> ped painting with the brush and had begun painting with his fingers
> directly on the canvas and seemed unable to stop. In reviewing the situa-
> tion with him, it became clear that to refuse to allow him to use this
> medium would only create more frustration and reinforce his feelings of
> inadequacy. Therefore, it was suggested that he conceptualize his ideas
> first in pastels on paper, then copy his own drawing in oil paint. In this
> way, he established some structure thus avoiding regression and fulfilling
> his wish to progress to a more difficult medium (Levick, 1975, p. 94).

Many mental patients who have been hospitalized for years have
learned that doing something is good for them. Art therapy can provide an activity that may alleviate anxiety. In this art activity, ver-
balization may not be elicited and is, in fact, not necessary. Gratification is obtained from the act of participating in the creative process. In effect, the gratification stimulates better social adaptation
and provides opportunity for further development in this area. It
also provides a form of re-socialization for the chronic patient who
often feels isolated from society.

The involutional-depressed patient usually resists any request to
perform a task that might reflect his/her feelings of helplessness and
inadequacy. Therefore, the art therapist must be cognizant of this
and not offer any activity or project that would cause frustration or
anxiety. The art therapist must keep in mind, too, that if electroconvulsive therapy (ECT) is given, there will be a transitory memory
loss. Hence, to engage a patient who has been given ECT in any activity should foster ego enhancement. One ECT patient, encouraged
to draw or paint anything he wanted with the art therapist acting as
teacher, obtained considerable gratification from the experience.
Having no conscious awareness of hostile feelings, he projected these
onto a painting of a ferocious fish, which he proudly carried home
with him when he was discharged from the hospital (Levick, 1975).
Thus, he was able to externalize these feelings through socially acceptable creative expression.

Obsessive–compulsive, neurotic patients rely heavily on their
ability to intellectualize and often resist involvement in an activity,
particularly a non-verbal one such as drawing or painting. Here,
too, the art therapist must be skilled in therapeutic techniques in

order to establish a therapeutic relationship. It is sometimes helpful to draw with this type of patient and to project thoughts and ideas onto the same piece of paper in a shared experience. Mirroring as a means of confrontation can be particularly useful here. For example, a young woman reported a dream and, when asked how she felt upon awakening, said she was very depressed. The art therapist asked her to draw these feelings; the patient took brush in hand, dipped into the paint, and furiously put strokes of vivid color across the paper. The art therapist proceeded to mirror this demonstration and then asked the patient to describe the therapist's actions and product. The patient could not avoid recognizing that this reflected anger, not depression, and had to own up to this feeling for herself even though it was still somewhat removed from conscious awareness. These kinds of interactions cut through lengthy obsessive verbalizations and facilitate the ability of the patient with this disorder to get in touch with feelings that can then be expressed.

There are numerous articles in the literature describing work with alcoholics, prisoners and children, both physically and emotionally handicapped. A great deal of work has been done with families, particularly using the art therapy evaluation designed by Kwiatkowska many years ago. This evaluation is used widely throughout the country by art therapists working with different kinds of populations, both child and adult. The evaluation consists of six tasks (Kwiatkowska, 1967, pp. 52-69) and provides a considerable amount of data about individual ego strengths and weaknesses and family interactions. Often, data elicited through the art therapy evaluation will provide direction for future therapeutic interventions.

Some time ago a request was made to this author to evaluate a family facing the problem of dealing with the terminal illness of a nineteen-year-old son. The young man, whose illness had been discovered when he was fourteen, had had his leg amputated and been given a prosthesis which he handled very well. In the evaluation, the parents and children (son and daughter, aged 23) were asked to represent family members. The father, who had originally protested that he could not draw but was finally persuaded to express himself as best he could on paper, drew family members, all without completed lower limbs. During the evaluation, this and other sensitive issues were not pointed out. However, when the family recognized the need for therapy after reviewing evaluation with the therapist, the father's drawing of the family suggested the direction of the therapeutic process not just for the father but for the entire family. It had become obvious that one way of denying their son's illness was for the parents to act as if they too had physical problems, and this was initially manifested in the father's representation of all family members with incomplete lower limbs.

Greater awareness of learning disabilities on the part of educators has reinforced early writings by Kramer (1958) and Naumburg (1966) regarding the knowledge that can be gained of developmental sequences and intrapsychic conflicts registered in children's drawings. They and other well-known art therapists have demonstrated that spontaneous drawings of both children and adults reveal normal and pathological evidence of fears, fantasies, thoughts, and affects, stimulated by internal and external pressures, ego strengths and weaknesses, id derivatives, and normal and abnormal defensive mechanisms (Levick, Dulicai, Briggs, and Billock, 1979).

Through the use of children's drawings, the trained art therapist can guide the therapeutic team in pinpointing developmental, motoric, perceptual, or emotional problems that may interfere with learning" (Levick et al., 1979, p. 364).

There is little in the published literature regarding the use of art therapy with children, but in the reference cited (i.e. Levick et al., 1979) there is a list of unpublished theses that do address this problem from several differing viewpoints. The reader is also referred to the bibliography listed at the end of this book and particularly to *Art Therapy: A Bibliography* (Gantt & Strauss, 1974).

Summary

In terms of a body of literature and scientific documentation, art therapy is a young profession. As more and more graduate students are required to write theses as part of their programs, it is hoped that they will answer the need for more scientific documentation. "The similarity between this methodology of art therapy and psychoanalytic psychology provides the art therapist with an enormous amount of clinical information which implies a greater appreciation for this modality as a diagnostic and therapeutic process" (Vaccaro, 1973).

There are those who have traditionally criticized the use of art as a vehicle for psychotherapy and feel that it should remain in the background of the mental health sciences as an *adjunctive therapy*. Zwerling (1979) addressed this issue with a question: "To which category of therapy do the (creative) art therapies belong?" His response clearly stated that this can be determined only by the context in which they are used. At different points in a program of treatment, different forms of psychotherapy may take center stage, and others may move from central to adjunctive position. Spurgeon English, in the foreword to his remarkable compilation of essays on a combined verbal and movement analysis of a psychotherapy session, states, "Events are incomprehensible except in terms of the context in which they occur" (in Zwerling, 1979).

As stated above, scientific documentation has not been forthcoming. The most valid documentation, however, is the picture made by the patient/client and translated appropriately by the trained and skilled art therapist. The art therapist can then help the patient/client to see and to understand the meaning of his graphic production, own it, and either accept or change the discovered emotional content towards self-awareness and growth. This modality, even when used in conjunction with other psychotherapies, contributes to the therapeutic process beyond that which is generally attributed to an adjunctive therapy. The field of art therapy has grown from the efforts of a very small group of pioneers, who from different educational, geographic backgrounds eventually communicated with each other and so many others, to demonstrate that which Anna Freud said to Erik Erikson, "Psychoanalysis may need people who make others see" (Coles, 1970).

In the chapter which will discuss aspects of psychosexual and cognitive development manifested in drawings, further examples of the relationship between psychoanalytic psychology and art therapy will be reviewed briefly.

Chapter Two

DEFENSE MECHANISMS OF THE EGO:
A DEVELOPMENTAL PERSPECTIVE

THE scope of this book does not allow for a comprehensive review of the literature on the subject of defense mechanisms, but an overview of the various defenses first described by Sigmund Freud will be presented. More attention will be paid to the literature that (1) relates a defense mechanism to a certain level of development and (2) reflects an adaptive or maladaptive process to reality. This will serve as a basis for the further understanding of the relationship of defense mechanisms to cognitive and psychosexual development as they are manifested in drawings.

Historical Overview

During the years 1893 to 1894, Sigmund Freud directed his investigations to the problems of neuroses (Rothgeb, 1972). In an early paper on the neuro-psychoses of defense, Sigmund Freud (1894) described theoretical ideas that formed the basis for all of his later work. The concept of defense mechanisms of the ego emerged from his examination of symptom formations tied to specific emotional disorders such as phobias, obsessions, and the syndrome of hysteria. While the conflicts producing these symptoms were described in relationship to specific developmental issues, the original definition of defenses was not discussed along decisive developmental lines.

Sigmund Freud reported two cases in which the defense against an incompatible idea was to separate that idea from its affect. While the idea remained conscious, it was isolated from the accompanying affect (i.e. isolation of affect). He described a situation in which the ego rejects both the incompatible idea and its affect to the degree that the individual "behaved as if the idea never occurred" and psychosis is imminent. At that time, he proposed a working hypothesis for the neurosis of defense, which stated, "In mental functions something is to be distinguished (quota of affect or sum of excitation) which possess all the characteristics of a quantity which is capable of increase,

16

diminution, displacement and discharge, and which is spread over the memory traces of ideas" (Sigmund Freud, 1894, in Rothbeg, 1972, p. 23).

Repression, described as both a theory and a defense, was designated by Sigmund Freud (1894) as the cornerstone for the whole structure of psychoanalysis. In 1921, he mentioned *projection* in his discussion of animism, magic, and omnipotence of thoughts. He said man uses the ideas of demons and spirits to project his own emotional impulses (Sigmund Freud, in Rothgeb, 1972).

Later papers by Sigmund Freud described regression as a successful ego defense against the demands of the libido. He further noted that in obsessional cases more than in normal and hysterical ones, the castration complex motivated employment of such defenses as reaction formation, undoing, regression, and isolation (1926, in Rothgeb, 1972).

The defenses mentioned above continue to be elaborated on in the texts of Sigmund Freud's numerous writings. Further definitions of these and other defenses are given in *An Outline of Psychoanalysis* (Sigmund Freud, 1940) and will be stated below.

According to Sigmund Freud, "instincts can change their aim" (p. 5). This is accomplished through the process of *displacement*. An example is repressed urges employed in the ego "undergoing sublimation with a displacement of the aims" (p. 12). *Identification* (as a defense) is described as "the most obvious reaction" to "replace . . . from within" a lost love object (p. 50). This process is discussed at length in relation to the Oedipal conflict (Sigmund Freud, 1940, pp. 47–50). *Regression* (i.e. a harkening back of the libido to "its earlier pregenital cathexes") occurs when the internal and/or the real external world present difficulties which precipitate a weakening of the ego (Sigmund Freud, 1940, p. 13).

It must be remembered that a good part of psychoanalytic theory took form from the reconstructions of the early childhood experiences of the neurotic and psychotic patients in treatment with Sigmund Freud. Observation of defense mechanisms was incorporated into the task of analysis, which is to learn as much as possible about the id, ego, and superego and their interactions with each other and the outside world (Anna Freud, 1936, rev. 1966). In analysis, the ego is perceived as the "seat of observation," and one of the goals of analysis is to explore the contents, boundaries, and functions of the ego. It is the ego through which knowledge of the id and superego is obtained. Id derivatives become apparent only when instinctual impulses are not gratified through transformations and feelings of tension and unpleasure are felt. In well-adapted individuals, boundaries between ego and superego are not easily differentiated. However, if guilt is evoked, observed superego criticism is perceived as the cause (Anna Freud, 1966). In the process of analysis, defensive measures against the id are unconscious and reconstructed in retrospect. Anna Freud also points out that chronological classifications of defense mechanisms are as uncertain as any "chronological pronouncements in analysis" (p. 53). She suggests that it would be more useful to study those situations in detail which invoke defensive reactions. However, it would seem to follow that if these situations can be identified as developmentally related there is a basis for conceptualizing a developmental perspective. It could also be assumed that, in addition to normal play and observable behavior, image formation of children and disturbed adults can reflect the development and utilization of the coping styles of well-adapted adults; minimal anxiety, stability, and flexibility would indicate that such mechanisms as repression and reaction formation, among others, are effectively functioning. It is proposed here that both adaptive and maladaptive defense mechanisms are manifested in spontaneous drawings of children and adults and will serve as an index of ego function.

For example, successful repression becomes known only "when it becomes apparent that something is missing" (Anna Freud, 1966, p. 8). Another example is *reaction formation*, which is an important defense adopted by the ego against the id. Analytic observation could easily view this as a spontaneous development of the ego, but distinct manifestations of obsessional behavior indicate that it is reaction initiated to conceal a long-standing conflict (Anna Freud, 1966). It is important to recognize that the process of repression is revealed in neurosis when "repressed material returns and reaction formations are revealed in the process of disintegration" (Anna Freud, 1966, p. 9).

In discussing neurotic symptoms, Anna Freud (1966) describes a consistent relationship between certain neuroses and a particular "mode of defense." She connects repression with hysteria, and isolation and undoing with obsessional neurosis. In the case of hysterical patients, conflict is centered around sexual impulses, and the need to repress these leads to symptom formation. The obsessional patient isolates "ideas from affects" and makes no connection between some thought and feeling. The need to maintain this separation often leads to obsessional ruminations and ritualistic behavior. Some other defense mechanisms described by Anna Freud (1966), and based on the earlier works of Sigmund Freud (1915, 1922), include introjection, identification, projection, reversal, and turning against the self. As these are illustrated, their function will be discussed.

An analogy is made between infantile neuroses and adult neuroses in terms of defenses. In both situations, anxiety states demand attention from the ego. Defense against anxiety in both cases is engaged by the ego because of an awareness that the instinct is dangerous since gratification has been forbidden by the caretakers in the case of the child and the restrictive superego in the case of the adult. Therefore, it is anxiety in the child and adult that is the motivating force underlying defensive processes. As the adult ego strives for synthesis, pleasure experienced in gratifying an instinct would be followed by unpleasure emanating from feelings of guilt; similarly, the child would fear abandonment or loss of love, and later punishment from the outside world. The reality of the individual's world, as it has been perceived through developmental phases, shapes the nature of the defensive process. This defensive process in the well-adapted adult evolves concomitantly with the reality process. The same process holds true for defenses against affects associated with instincts regardless of whether those affects are pleasurable or unpleasurable. Those defenses employed by children "which are governed simply by the pleasure principle are themselves more primitive in character" (Anna Freud, rev. 1966, p. 62). It would appear then that understanding defenses, in terms of the pleasure versus reality principle, would also serve as an aid in placing them along developmental lines in the "normal" child and adult and aid in identifying conflicted areas of development for the disturbed child or adult.

As noted above, when Anna Freud first wrote about defense mechanisms (1936), she defined them in a somewhat chronological order but focused more on their use in certain situations. She felt at that time that a chronological order was not consistent with clinical observations of children manifesting neurotic symptoms. In her later work (Anna Freud 1965) and prior to the revision of her first work (1966), she expands on her original viewpoint and prefers not to differentiate between defense and adaptation, nor to describe defenses as either pathological or normal. She prefers instead to make a distinction between different results obtained by their use and describes four factors on which these results depend. A chronological order is strongly supported.

For the first factor, "age adequateness," she states that the chronology of defenses is an approximate one, and if they are used before the appropriate age or employed for an extended period after that age, they are likely to produce pathological results. Denial and projection, "normal" in childhood, if continued in the late adolescent or adult, can lead to pathology. Likewise, repression and reaction formation, if "used too early," may have a crippling effect on the child's personality.

The second factor, "balance," implies that a healthy organization exists when the ego has at its disposal more than one defense mechanism and employs different methods to deal with "various danger situations arising from the id" (Anna Freud, 1965, p. 177).

"Intensity," the third factor, is concerned with the quantitative versus qualitative aspects of defenses. It is the quantity, rather than the quality, of utilization of a defense which determines whether the defense "leads to symptom formation" or "healthy social adaptation." "Reversibility," the fourth factor, is also essential for adaptation. For example, if an individual continues to deal with past anxieties related to dangers that no longer exist, appropriate reversibility has not occurred. This may be an indication of pathology (Anna Freud, 1965).

These factors are critical aspects of the Metapsychological Profile, an approach to diagnostic assessment outlined by Anna Freud (1965). In a future effort it is being planned to correlate and contrast the Metapsychological Profile and Art Therapy Evaluation as diagnostic assessments.

Chronological Development of Defenses

In spite of some obvious unease with the notion of a chronological classification, Anna Freud does place defenses tentatively at certain stages of development. This is strongly supported by other investigators, including Kestenberg (1975) and Greenspan (1979).

Oral Stage (0–18 Months)

Kestenberg (1975) describes two types of early defenses related to early fears. The first, inhibition of impulses, is discussed in terms of both normal and pathological precursors of social adaptations. On the one hand, while serving as an effective protection of the self, it may also inhibit function. Conversely, to some degree it may be useful in aiding the child to develop realistic behaviors that lead to social consideration of others. The second, motor discharge, is increased under stress. Both defenses, according to Kestenberg, originate in infancy and are related to the interaction between child and caretaker. The child quickly learns to recognize disapproval and early on will inhibit impulses that evoke such disapproval. Crying, an example of motor discharge, and initially a "reflex-like action," develops into "a signal of distress," but where that distress is not responded to may become experienced as the only means of relief (Kestenberg, 1975).

Kestenberg believes that both inhibition and motor discharge "are basic attitudes upon which a superstructure of defensive and non-defensive coping mechanisms are built" (1975, p. 188). In the process of delaying, diminishing, or assisting in reversing the "impact or course of movement," inhibition "becomes the motor counterpart and model for reaction formation, denial, isolation, repression and intellectualization" (p. 188). She cites Fenichel (1928) and goes on to connect inhibition as an underlying force in the development of concentrated attention and internalization. Of motor discharge, she believes that on a continuum it is the basis for "such mechanisms as displacement, turning from passivity to activity, acting out, identification with the aggressor, as well as coping with reality and externalization" (Kestenberg, 1975, p. 188).

Greenspan (1979) states that along developmental lines primary process employs "displacement, condensation and substitute formation" (p. 121).

Anal Stage (18–36 Months)

Regression, reversal, or turning around on the self, although not clearly connected to a specific stage of development of the psychic structure, may be "the very earliest defense mechanisms employed by the ego" (Anna Freud, rev. 1966). Denial as a defense is used normally by children through fantasy, and this process allows the emerging ego to deny painful reality stimulated by sources of objective anxiety. The persistence of denial of reality in adult life may be indicative of a serious mental disorder. Children also use denial in "words and act," but, if overly supported by the adults in the child's environment, this may be a precursor to obsessional rituals (Anna Freud, rev. 1966). Introjection of the anxiety-producing object may manifest itself in what Anna Freud describes as "identification with the aggressor." In the process of impersonating the aggressor, imitating the aggression, the role of the victim is reversed, and in this sense projection as well as introjection is employed. Again, this may be considered normal when used by children to deal with conflicts connected to authority but can become pathological when carried over to adult personal relations. Projection, which is naturally used by children, is like repression in that it keeps instinctual processes from becoming perceived. An example of how this defense may be utilized is described above in relation to Sigmund Freud's ideas about demons and spirits reflecting man's projection of emotional impulses.

Anna Freud, in describing the development of the ego as a "product of the conflict," points out that the task of mastery in the very young child contributes to the development of the ego. During this period, the methods of defense reflect the influence of objective anxiety and ways to master this anxiety emerge (1966). The projection of these anxieties in graphic productions of children often serves as a form of mastery. This process will be discussed in the presentation of children's drawings in Chapter Four.

Oedipal Stage (3–5 Years)

In the Oedipal stage, children continue to use denial and also manifest avoidance, displacement, and condensation. Greenspan states these latter defenses emerge in the rapprochement subphase of separation individuation (18 months) and cites the work in this area by Mahler (1968). In this early pre-Oedipal stage, regression to an earlier mode of relating and functioning may occur. Greenspan

(1979) attributes the phenomenon to this rapprochement subphase, resulting from a lack of sufficient emotional support from nurturing caretaker(s), and refers here to the work of Mahler, Pine, and Bergman (1975).

Discussing projection, he refers to Sigmund Freud's explanation of animism and its relation to this defense in dealing with some emotions. Like early man, children seek to control the world around them and to this end employ magical thinking. This incorporates an "animistic mode of thinking" in which the children's emotional impulses are projected onto objects in the environment as if they were real (Sigmund Freud, in Rothgeb, 1972).

Post-Oedipal Stage (5–7 Years) *

The defense mechanisms of imitation, identification, and introjection are used by the ego "before, during and after the Oedipus complex." While they are necessary in preparation for future adaptation and foster internalization of parental values, etc., by themselves they do not insure this adaptation will be achieved (Anna Freud, 1965, p. 9). However, further into her work, Anna Freud states that the ability of a child's ego to deal with anxiety influences predictions regarding "future mental health or illness" (p. 136). She believes there is a better chance for mental health if children master danger rather than retreat from it. Incorporated into the process of mastery are those ego resources of "intellectual understanding, logical reasoning, changing of external circumstances, aggressive counterattack" (p. 136).

Identification is not only a defense employed during this period but is a major task. Successful repression of the infantile neuroses and the Oedipus complex is a crucial factor in this process of identification.

In order for repression to be employed by the ego, it must be assumed that the ego is no longer merged with the id; projection and introjection imply differentiation between ego (as it relates to self)

---

* This age period is most often described in the literature as "early latency." It is identified here as the post-Oedipal phase of development and will be so identified throughout the text. This author believes most children are still dealing with the tasks of the Oedipal period during the years five through seven, and the drawings produced by children at this time frequently support this. Some examples are provided in Chapter Four.

and outside world (Anna Freud, 1965). Greenspan also addresses this stage of development and points out that the relationship between the ego and reality is the focus of the "adaptive perspective" and cites Rappaport (1959) who suggests that reality plays a defensive conflictual role and influences the formation of ego structure in the process of identification with objects of social reality. He also states that in the pre-latency child, a certain amount of regression would be normal, while the degree of regression in an adult would be significant in making a diagnosis. Consistent with psychoanalytic theory, he describes the process of identification as critical in resolving the Oedipal conflict, and he observes that the nature of introjects determines the development of the superego (Greenspan, 1979).

Latency (7–11 Years)

Defenses reflect Oedipal derivatives, and an example would be the latency child who uses reaction formation to deal with superego restrictions emanating from the Oedipus complex and feelings of rage. In addition, Greenspan (1979) views the early latency period as a time to try to see the development of individual defenses. Regression to the pre-Oedipal period vis-à-vis splitting of good and bad (mother, father, siblings, etc.) would be an indicator of unresolved phases of development. This would suggest that some pre-Oedipal conflict had not been resolved, successful repression was not present, and anxiety from instinctual drives was interfering with intellectual pursuits. Conversely, identification connotes a resolution of Oedipal conflict. In the case of a boy who has a positive male identity, this would indicate the resolution of rage toward the father. If there is no resolution or the resolution is negative (i.e. identification with the parent of the opposite sex), magical thinking, and primitive defenses, such as denial, avoidance, etc., will persist. Phase-specific defensive operations of the ego (i.e. reaction formation and rationalization) reinforce repression in the latency period, allowing the child to address the developmental tasks of that period.

Rappaport (1951b, in Greenspan, 1979) described rationalization as a defense that takes place when secondary process thinking needs to compromise prohibited drive goals with superego restrictions and the outside world. Of the intellectualization process he believes we know only a little; as a defense it is related to autonomous functions of the ego and is thinking which, while using drive energy, remains unconflicted by it. Developmentally, the normal latency child has obsessive defensive patterns to keep fantasies repressed, which is consistent with the analytic construct that at this phase of development successful repression frees the ego to pursue and relate to the outside world (Greenspan, 1979).

Adolescence and Beyond

Greenspan (1979) describes the mature person as one who, through the process of identification, has been able to integrate concepts of "different self and object representations from different stages of childhood and adolescence with real perceptions of external social environment, as well as with ideals, values and expectations of the future" (p. 68). Another important process is the capacity to neutralize drive energy and transform drive derivatives into socially acceptable activities. The defenses of displacement and reaction formation along with neutralization lead to adaptive transformations (Greenspan, 1979). He also defines the healthy individual as one who, when in touch with the "self," can experience a wide range of feelings, can reverse actions in thought, and can also integrate opposite feelings such as love and hate for the same person. This is consistent with Anna Freud's (1966) factor of reversibility and supports the notion of the capacity of the flexible ego to utilize different defense mechanisms for different situations.

Though the population referred to in this work, in terms of normal adaptive manifestations of defenses in drawings, is two to ten years of age, it may be useful to cite some literature on the abnormal manifestations of defenses in disturbed adolescents and adults as these will be illustrated also. An adolescent who has not worked through the Oedipus complex and its accompanying castration anxiety may use avoidance both in thought and action. Shunning of intellectual and physical pursuits that threaten masculinity is an example of avoidance, and Greenspan (1979) writes of the adolescent boy who avoids members of the opposite sex. Used to excess, these maneuvers can inhibit those tasks that need to be accomplished for successful transition to adulthood. Greenspan also cites Zetzel (1968), who purports that defenses utilized in hysterical behaviors are related to issues emanating from a less "developmentally advanced organization." A discussion of hysterical symptoms in Moore and Fine (1968) places these issues at the Oedipal period and reports them as resulting from difficulty in resolving the Oedipal conflict. The two major defenses, according to them, are repression and regression, leading to "hysterical symptoms" related to body parts and affects.

Where repression pushes dangerous instincts back into the id and keeps "ideational representatives" unconscious, projection displaces "into the outside world." This can be a debilitating defense when, for example, feelings of jealousy and aggressive behavior are projected onto another. In a more healthy process, the combination of projection and identification, when used for defensive purposes, can gratify an individual's own instinctual wishes through fulfillment of someone else's wishes and fantasies and can even lead to becoming the champion of someone else's rights. Anna Freud (1966) describes this as "altruistic surrender." There are excellent examples of these defensive maneuvers throughout Anna Freud's work. The reader is referred to her writing for a more comprehensive treatment of the subject.

Throughout the years, many psychologists, psychiatrists, and mental health professionals have been concerned with ego functions and have addressed this enormous subject from many different perspectives. Some of those viewpoints specifically related to defense mechanisms and their place in the developmental sequence will be presented.

Anna Freud suggests that the "nature of the psychic structure in childhood and latency" (1966, p. 149) is crucial in determining the course of adolescence. A number of relative factors decide the resolution of the adolescent upheaval. Among these is the choice of defense mechanisms that the ego can call on and their efficiency in dealing with various types of anxiety to maintain equilibrium. She also points out that these will vary according to the different constitutional factors and developmental lines within individuals. The significance of the effect of constitutional factors and individual developmental lines in the early years on healthy adaptation has been evident throughout this author's clinical experience and was a determining factor in deciding to focus on the years of growth between the ages of two and ten in this work. Although it is not presumed that the personality structure observable during those years is sufficient to determine the outcome of adolescence and passage into adulthood, it is believed that it is possible to identify strength and weakness through the knowledge of defense mechanisms utilized in drawings and how they reflect other aspects of critical developmental issues. This information can provide further data in assessing the capacities of the ego to handle the normal developmental stresses. According to Anna Freud, the ego is "victorious" when defensive measures successfully deal with anxiety, provide "some measure of gratification," and establish "the most harmonious relations possible between the id, the superego and the forces of the outside world" (1966, p. 176).

Greenspan states his own clinical view of defenses as that they range from "optimal to less optimal" (1979, p. 282). Categorizing them developmentally, he places projection and introjection on a primitive level and intellectualization on the most advanced level. Characteristics of defenses include stability, flexibility, selectivity, and effectiveness (1979). These are similar to the factors listed above by Anna Freud (1965). Greenspan believes defenses have the greatest field of application and mobility when they "can deal with a wide range of stimuli (drive and affects) and can move between advanced and less advanced states in a selective manner" (p. 282). His concept for an intact ego requires that the "basic ego apparatuses and basic ego functions" be capable of performing those tasks (in Piagetian terms) of the concrete operational stage (p. 290). This stage usually begins around six or seven years of age and continues until ten or eleven years and suggests to this author (in analytic terms) that, in the well-functioning child, the Oedipal situation and normal developmental conflicts from oral and anal phases of development have been appropriately defended against, freeing the child to address the tasks of learning and making peer relationships.

In Rappaport's view, thought organization emerges from developmental motivational and defensive dynamics of the ego (1951b). He relates defenses to communication and sees them as limiting communications, which can enrich ego function and aid in solving problems, achieving gratification of drives consonant with the reality principle, and synthesizing internal and external systems. In this sense, Rappaport (in Greenspan, 1979) seems to be separating communication from defenses that are maladaptive. Noting Anna

Freud's (1965) concept of defenses and adaptation, well-adapted individuals would employ defenses that would support communication as Rappaport describes. Another concept of communication in relation to the defenses must be noted as it pertains to this work, that is, defenses, whether adaptive or maladaptive, whether enhancing or limiting ego function by themselves, serve as communication about personality development. The degree to which they are used and the circumstances that evoke particular defensive activity "communicate" something about the style of an individual's thinking and coping.

Summary

In this chapter, the early work of Sigmund and Anna Freud pertaining to defense mechanisms as a function of the ego has been briefly reviewed, with a specific focus on developmental relationships. Their description of these phenomena is rooted in that part of psychoanalytic theory that pertains to the interaction of id, ego, and superego in which the role of defense mechanisms is to bind the anxiety produced by internal and/or external conflicts. While initially seen as a pathological phenomenon, their view of defenses binding anxiety was later changed to one in which defense mechanisms, as an element in the process of development, may lead to adaptive as well as to maladaptive behaviors. The original perspective also described defenses primarily observed in those situations in which their use could be understood in relation to the neuroses. Ms. Freud expanded on this, and in her later work discusses defenses in relation to developmental stages.

This relationship is further defined by others cited above, including Rappaport, Zetzel, and Greenspan. Though not in total agreement, they do concur to the degree that beginnings of a developmental hierarchy of ego defense mechanisms can be recognized. They also generally agree that by late latency the well-adapted individual would have available defenses that could selectively deal with a wide range of stimuli.

This chapter has dealt primarily with psychoanalytic theory related to defense mechanisms, and little correlation to Piagetian theory other than the one just noted has been made. Up to now, these correlations have been deliberately avoided, and the intent has been to prepare the reader with an introduction to psychoanalytic concepts which form the basis of this work. However, the overall intent is to illustrate developmental relationships between psychosexual development and cognitive development through the identification of defense mechanisms in children's drawings.

Developmental stages of cognitive skills (according to Piaget), a general overview of psychosexual development and developmental sequences in children's drawings will be correlated in the following chapter.

Chapter Three

PSYCHOSEXUAL AND COGNITIVE DEVELOPMENT: THEIR RELATIONSHIP TO DEVELOPMENTAL SEQUENCES IN CHILDREN'S DRAWINGS: A THEORETICAL OVERVIEW

FEW developmental psychologists would dispute that Freud and Piaget have laid the groundwork for understanding cognitive and psychosexual development. Gardner (1973) points out that Freud emphasizes the personality and the emotional life of the individual and the relationship "between psychosexual experience and cognitive processes." Piaget, on the other hand, is interested primarily in those mental processes that result in scientific thought and can be expressed in logical terms. Gardner (1973) suggests that the only way to understand a holistic view of human development is to psychologically analyze the arts and the artist. His frame of reference for this is collectively "the artist, audience member, performer and critic." However, a basic problem lies in the fundamental differences between the theories of Sigmund Freud and Piaget. Sigmund Freud viewed the oral, anal, and phallic phases as sequences that often overlap. Piaget defines structured stages, each one having distinct characteristics. An example of this would be the "systematic and well-integrated network of logical structures" ascribed to the concrete operational stage "in contrast to the preoperational period which is unsystematic" (Rosen, 1972, p. 26). Piaget does not see *affectivity* as a condition in structure formation (Piaget, 1962). He postulates that cognitive factors can ameliorate affective difficulties, but concurs with Freud that there is no "purely affective state" or "purely cognitive state." He views them as parallel and describes affect as the force in behavior, and the structure as cognitive.

In order to "structure" (my word) his concept of this parallel, he equates moral values with conservation of values, "will" (i.e. "affective operation") is regarded equal to cognitive operation in the concrete operational stage and "personality," which he believes emerges in the formal operational stage, representing the "Superior Synthesis of Affective Life" (Piaget, 1951).

There have been numerous studies to support Piaget's stage theory, but Smedsland (1969) and Flavell (1972) have suggested cognitive–developmental sequences and the recognition of a relationship between all mental processes and the meaning of the subject's acts.

In the process of preparing the most efficient, yet comprehensive way to present this correlative overview, a considerable amount of related literature has been omitted. While determining what to include, I was reminded of the problem one faces when presented with an array of delectable appetizers, knowing an enormous dinner is to follow. Consequently, the choices were made to prepare the way for what will follow. To aid the reader interested in pursuing this area, a general bibliography is given.

Piagetian Theory

In keeping with the decision stated, this will be a brief overview. Further elaboration of specific stages will be incorporated with discussion of children's drawings in the following chapter, and a list of Piagetian terminology is defined in the Glossary. Rosen (1978) discusses Piaget's work in a format useful to clinicians, developmentalists, and educators and will be the major source of information for this theory of cognitive development.

The method employed in Piaget's research is direct observation, with a significant emphasis on discussions between investigator and child. This is not a standardized aproach, and the investigator must take cues from the child he is observing. There are four major developmental periods. The first, the sensorimotor period, is from zero to two years of age and is "characterized by a profound egocentrism" (Rosen, 1978, p. 11). This period is marked as the basis and root of Piaget's theoretical construct of development skills. In the early stage of infancy, there is no differentiation between self and outside world. All actions engaged in by the child "tend to be body centered" (p. 11). There is a gradual lessening of the involvement with self (egocentrism) and a progressive awareness of other objects in the environment as separate from himself. During this process, intelligent behavior is marked by the "adaptation of a means to achieve an end" (p. 11) and proceeds from "accidental manipulation upon the environment" to deliberate action (Rosen, 1978). Piaget's view that intelligence develops from the child's actions upon his environment is critical in understanding the difference between this developmental theory and Sigmund Freud's, which will be discussed further. An important function of this period is a growing knowledge of reality in terms of space, causality, time, and object permanence. The period is not specifically relevant to the observations of children's drawings for obvious reasons. Like psychosexual development, the development of cognition and intelligent behavior is dependent on and consistent with normal physiologic growth. Without normal motoric development, the child cannot act upon or move about in his environment. And until a child has achieved and mastered grasping reflexes (around 12–18 months), he would not be able to hold or guide a crayon or other graphic media. Therefore, it will be assumed that the drawings presented below and identified as produced by normal children reflect that the child has achieved normal motoric growth and is at the youngest (i.e. 18 months) age. Impairment in motoric growth, either genetically or as a result of an accident, has serious implications for both cognitive and psychosexual growth. Although beyond the scope of this work, some manifestations of organic problems in drawings will be presented in the section on images reflecting psychopathology. An important achievement of this period and of particular importance to the subject of this work is the ability to use symbols, which heralds the first phase of the next period (Rosen, 1978).

The pre-operational period, which extends from approximately two to seven years of age, is marked by both a static quality and a movement towards representation. Thinking is not yet part of an organized structure. The symbolic function, later changed by Piaget to semiotic function, through its two components of signs and symbols allows the child to mentally represent past and future. The concept of symbolization is of major import here. Though signs and symbols like those used in mathematics and science become part of socially shared knowledge, it is the private symbol connected to dreams and "mental images, symbolic play and deferred imitation" (Piaget, 1946/1962, in Rosen, 1978) that have bearing on the production of graphic images. Both symbols and signs represent objects which are "not present to the perceptual apparatus" (p. 13). Symbols, however, in addition to being private, are motivated and "tend to be ego-involved" (p. 13). An important difference between a symbol and a sign is that a symbol resembles the absent object it signifies in some way. Rosen cites Furth (1966), who interprets Piaget's use of the term "symbolic" as more closely related to the Freudian concept of symbol than to "symbolic–logic" (1978). Therefore, the term "symbolic" carries with it an "element of egocentrism" insofar as it does not reflect "objective comprehension" anticipated in advanced logical thinking processes (Rosen, 1978). This period should be of particular interest to clinicians in that it includes language and thought development, along with "modes of reasoning," the child's view of the world and causality, and the process of the child's moral development. Piaget, in his early works, describes these areas of achievement more in terms of limitation than mastery, but knowledge of this period lays the groundwork for a better understanding of further development in the domain of cognition.

Rosen points out that, although there is a considerable lessening of egocentric behavior during this period, the child's thinking remains centered, and he is still unable to attend to "two or more aspects simultaneously." The ability to decenter his thinking and not be misled by visual cues occurs later, enabling him to process information "in a more accurate and adaptive fashion" (1978, p. 14). One other important characteristic of this period is the concept of irreversibility. While the child at this time is able to follow a process from its beginning to its end, he cannot retrace his steps to the starting point of that process, regardless of whether it is a simple or complex procedure. Because of its relevance to mental representations and imagery and symbolic formation, the child's view of the world during this time is characterized by animism, realism, artificialism, and participation (See the Glossary of Piagetian terms at the back of this book for definitions of these concepts). During the later part of the pre-operational period, the child "moves from centering on states toward comprehending transformations . . ., thinking becomes semireversible," and a more mature approach to conceptualization becomes apparent (Rosen, 1978, p. 15).

The third period, identified as the concrete operational period, begins at approximately age six or seven years and extends over the next five or six years. The child can now recognize groupings of classifications and seriate. This capacity leads to more highly organized and systematic thought processes. The term *concrete* is applied to operations because "they apply to objects and not verbal hypotheses" (p. 18). Lewis (1963) interprets this to mean that the child is not free to examine or hypothesize about absent or present abstract relationships, and thought processes are primarily connected to actual aspects of a given situation (Rosen, 1978). However, thinking is no longer centered; the capacity to reverse procedures is available. Conservation (the ability to recognize that some properties of an object, in spite of certain modifications, remain the same), not seen in the preoperational period, develops here. The facility to produce mental representations of familiar objects, whether they are present or not in the environment, is a particularly important fact in understanding and interpreting children's drawings produced during these years. The way in which they are produced in terms of drawing skills consistent with this age group, and the relationship of the images as mental representations to psychosexual development will be discussed and illustrated.

The formal operational period is the fourth and final developmental stage in Piaget's theory of cognition. Beginning at approximately eleven years of age and continuing until about fifteen years of age, the period is predominated by the awareness of the possible, beyond reality. Inhelder and Piaget (1955/1958, in Rosen, 1978) describe formal thinking as that which allows the adolescent to formulate hypotheses about facts and events regardless of whether or not they actually take place. The individual reaching this level is capable of conceptualizing and implementing scientific methodology. Reasoning is no longer tied to actual content, and the relationship between propositions can be addressed. Rosen points out that "the achievement of formal operations is not predetermined" (p. 23) and therefore not everyone attains this ability. He further reports that studies with some primitive tribes seem to indicate that within the entire group no adult member demonstrated the capacity for formal operational thinking.

As stated earlier, this study on defense mechanisms manifested in drawings deals with a normal population of approximately two to ten years of age, and the stage of formal operations will not be probed. It will be indicated that authorities in the fields of cognitive and psychosexual theory seem to agree that the most critical periods of development leading to a mature adaptation are those preceding the fourth period. Concomitant with this, illustrations in the section on psychopathology will show that there is little evidence of formal operational thinking in the drawings of adult psychotic patients and no evidence of it in those produced by disturbed adolescents.

There are some components of this theory of cognitive development that are germane to all four periods discussed above and also to psychoanalytic theory and the theory of art therapy presented in the next chapter. The reader is reminded that some of the terminology may be specific to Piaget and, for clarification, is referred again to the Glossary of Piagetian terms at the back of this book. Organization, a biological concept, is "essentially an internal matter" (Rosen, 1978, p. 7). Adaptation evolves through the developing relationship between the organism and external world. The interaction of the processes of assimilation and accommodation, both inherent in Piaget's theory, forms the basis for adaptation. Together they comprise the "most fundamental ingredients of intellectual functioning . . . present in every intellectual act" (p. 8). Rosen also points out, however, that this "relationship varies throughout development" (1978, p. 9). Assimilation predominates in play, whereas accommodation predominates in imitation. The image as a symbol is an "interiorization of previous perceptions. It is "personal or specific to the individual" producing it and its source lies in "material or sensorial properties of the object" even in the absence of that object (Rosen, 1978, p. 87). The progressive decline of egocentrism comes about as the result of peer social interaction during childhood. As this occurs, the child develops the capacity to evolve alternate views in the process of differentiating between his own and those of others. Rosen reports a study by Neale (1966) which demonstrated that disturbed children between the ages of eight and eleven years (hospitalized because of antisocial behavior in the community) were "significantly more egocentric" than the control group of normal children of the same age. This is important to keep in mind when reviewing the drawings of disturbed children in terms of the maladaptive defenses they employ and depict in their imagery.

Rosen's comprehensive review focused specifically on cognitive skills and current research in that area. However, it is clear that he supports the concept (a major focus of this presentation) that psychoanalysis be integrated with the work of the Geneva School (1978).

Piagetian and Psychoanalytic Theories:
A View Towards Integration

It was mentioned earlier that the idea for such an integration is neither unique nor recent. Wolff (1960, in Greenspan, 1979) examined the relationship between cognition and emotion in "human adaptation." However, according to Greenspan, Wolff did not develop "transformational bridges or functional relationships between emotion and intellect" (p. 2).

Piechowski (1975) reported that developmental psychology had produced no theory that included emotional development. Existing theories, he maintained, were either cognitive, ontogenetic, or both, and were all descriptive. His monograph describes a provocative theory originally developed by Kazimierz Dabrowski. In the foreword to Piechowski's monograph, Dabrowski describes his unwillingness to accept the idea of early childhood frustration as an explanation for the origin and development of psychoneuroses. In his clinical practice, he was impressed with the "creative and developmental richness" expressed by patients suffering from mental disorders and "especially psychoneuroses" (p. 236). From this, he perceived a link between the psychoneurotic and creative processes.

Dabrowski also rejected a "one-sided unilevel transposition of experimental results with animals carried out with Pavlovians or Behaviorists onto complex subtle and multi-level human mechanisms" (pp. 234–235). He perceived an outline of a hierarchy of values and was compelled to develop a "hierarchy of values which would be described with precision, empirically developed and objectively testable" (p. 235). Psychological and educational experiments revealed that in the area of education phenomena were multileveled. He does not believe that complex behavior of human life can be described without investigation of links, aggregations and interactions of factors operating in the external environment and inner psychic milieu. He points out that children who are sensitive and capable are often given negative evaluations because of their shyness and apparent lack of confidence. Cognitive as well as experiential potential made it possible for him to develop a multi-dimensional and multi-level construct that has bearing on the philosophy of education and development of educational models. He also sees it as useful for diagnosis and treatment of mental disorder. "A theory to claim generality must include emotional development and offer a means of explaining, rather than only describing, developmental transformation" (Dabrowski, in Piechowski, 1975, p. 239). Built on Jacksonian principles of evolution of levels of functioning, Dabrowski's theory of positive disintegration fulfills the criteria put forth by Piechowski above. In this theory, development is viewed as a function of behavioral organization. There are five levels, each with a distinct structure. The structure of a higher level replaces the structure of a lower one through the process of positive disintegration. Developmental patterns (DP) have observable dimensions of mental functioning. There are five mental functions that are identified as psychomotor, sensual, imaginational, intellectual, and emotional modes. The strength of these five modes of experiencing "advances and accelerates" the development of an individual (p. 256). A brief interpretation of these five modes follows.

"Psychomotor excitability" seems to emerge from an "organic excess of energy." It is manifested in "rapid talk, violent games," and "pressure for action" sometimes observed in delinquent behavior (p. 256). Distress may be converted into "gesticulation, pacing, throwing objects, wanderlust, . . . chain-smoking" (p. 257).

"Sensual overexcitability" reflects "heightened experiencing of sensory pleasure" and is manifested in a "need for comfort luxury" along with different sexual experiences and "superficial relationships" (p. 257). Overeating is one example of a "transfer of emotional tension."

"Imaginational overexcitability" produces rich associations of "images and impressions, inventiveness, use of image and metaphor in verbal expression, strong and sharp visualization" (p. 257). Here, emotional tension is "transferred to dreams, nightmares" as well as other "fearful expressions" (p. 257).

"Intellectual overexcitability" is manifested in the expression of continual curiosity (i.e. "avidity for knowledge, analysis, theoretical thinking . . ."). According to Piechowski, this mode does not "manifest the transfer of emotional tension" as the first three do. He suggests that when "intellectual and emotional processes of high intensity occur together" the two components can be separated (1975, p. 257).

"Emotional overexcitability" is a "function of experiencing emotional relationships," which may be attached to persons, living things or places. Manifestations include inhibition, excitation, strong affective memory, concern with death, fears, anxieties, depressions, feelings of loneliness, need for security, concern for others, exclusive relationships, difficulties of adjustment to new environments (Piechowski, 1975, p. 258).

A strong potential for development is present "if all, or almost all, forms of overexcitability are present." A high level of development is contingent on the presence of excitability. The emotional form must be the strongest if the highest level of development is to occur, whereas if the psychomotor and sensual forms are greater in strength than the others, development will be limited to the lowest level (Piechowski, 1975, p. 258).

Various stages of development are often dissimilar and appear unrelated if the succession is not known. To secure continuity and regularity of development, an underlying structure is necessary. A general theory of human development should direct the psychologist's view of human behavior as "progression of revolving behavioral patterns . . . which are an interplay of hereditary, environmental and conscious self-determining factors" (Piechowski, 1975, pp. 242-243). He makes a distinct comparison between Piagetian theory and positive disintegration. In the former, different stages proceed in an orderly fashion and are the product of the process of development. In the latter "development is a function of the level of organization" (p. 245). What emerges is a non-ontogenetic evolutionary pattern of individual growth, encompassing emotional and cognitive development and producing a structure of behavior. This structure determines the level of development. The process of development from lower to higher level of functioning is produced by instability, partial or complete disorganization of behavior. Therefore affective and cognitive functions are restructured and reorganized by positive disintegration. A new organization of higher level functions results after a breakdown of the lower level (Piechowski, 1975).

The concepts of "developmental structures, developmental potential and the characteristics by which they can be detected and measured" are unique to Dabrowski's theory. Three empirical tests of the theory were performed on data collected from "atomistic analysis of autobiographies," but these results will not be reported here.

In this theory there are distinct levels of development. A level is a specific developmental structure and differs from a stage which may represent a segment of a sequence. When a "level is attained," it is understood that a higher level structure has replaced a lower level structure.

Unilevel and multi-level structures of behavior and development form the specific concept of this theory.

> These structures are recognized by the presence or absence of characteristic processes of operations called dynamisms. Integration is interpreted in a new way. Primary integration is equated with the absence of developmental dynamism, hence with the absence of development. Secondary integration is the culmination of development, but not its cessation. Rather it is the synthesis and unification of developmental processes (Piechowski, 1975, p. 266).

Piechowski further suggests that through the application of this theory inner conflict leads to self-awareness which in turn leads to a choice and decision in relation to personal growth. Self-determination is possible, and an individual can rise above the limitations of social environment.

Training and clinical experience lead this author to reject Dabrowski's position in relation to early childhood frustration and neurosis. However, others have supported his idea about a "link" between the psychoneurotic and creative processes (Kubie, 1958; Nagera, 1967; Hatter, 1965) and it has been an intriguing subject for many investigators. This is certainly of particular interest to art therapists who facilitate the creative process for the purpose of self-awareness through expression in some form of art media, working with normal and disturbed populations. Dabrowski's concept of secondary integration is not unlike the psychoanalytic concept of secondary elaboration. Kris (1952) has written extensively on regression in the service of the ego as it pertains to the creative processes. For a work of art to be truly considered as such, primary process material is disguised by secondary process elaboration, and the final product represents an organized whole (Kris, 1952), which would include the five mental functions described by Dabrowski and parallel his construct of an autonomous factor. It is my impression that an individual capable of such function would have indeed developed highly adaptive defenses and the capacity for formal operational thinking. The study is an interesting one and is reported in detail because of its divergent viewpoint and the fact that, unlike most theoretical propositions, it has been tested empirically. It would be interesting to compare Piechowski's results with evaluations of drawings produced by the same populations in terms of level of adaptive mechanisms and cognitive functions.

The work of Greenspan (1979), referred to previously, is by far the most ambitious and comprehensive attempt to integrate Piagetian and psychoanalytic theory. Further references to his work here represent only a small portion of his presentation and were selected on the basis of relevance to this material. For elaboration and clarification, the reader is referred to the original source.

Greenspan's objective was to develop a new model that would integrate Piaget's developmental model with the "psychoanalytic approach for further understanding of human adaptation" (p. 2). In his view, a structural theory must "include a central construct and give account of the system's inherent laws of transformation" (p. 12). In a review of some previous efforts by Odier (1956), Cobliner (1967), Anthony (1956a), and Wolff (1960) to integrate these two theories, Greenspan concludes that both theories "hold that psychic energy is controlled by intrapsychic rather than physical agents" (p. 8). In addition, both theories describe a developmental sequence on a continuum of self-control from a lesser degree to a greater degree. He cites Kaplan (1972) who points out that specific features of one theory can be helpful "as an organizing principle" for information obtained from another theory. As an example, Kaplan suggests that content emanating from the analytic point of view (drive stimulus) may have bearing on the cognitive structures described as the "major organizing constructs" in the theory postulated by Piaget.

Greenspan (1979) reports many differences of opinion regarding the concept of mental representations, particularly in connection with learning theory. He implies that "mental representation" may signify a process of reconstructing a figurative image although an external stimulus is not present, and that in this sense "there is a virtual identity between Piaget's 'evocative memory' and psychoanalytic 'mental representation.'" Silverman (1971, in Greenspan) suggests that the transition from pre-logical to logical thinking (studied by Piaget) is parallel to the psychoanalytic concept of the transition from primary process to secondary process thinking. Holt (1967) discussed primary process from the perspective of Piaget's structuralism, but presented a divergent viewpoint. It was Holt's belief that the primary process is a separate "structural system in its own right." He bases this on the fact that "condensations, displacements involved in the construction of stable defenses, repetitiveness of dream elements, stability of neurotic symptoms and the universality of certain symbols" all support the notion that there is "a structural foundation and development to the primary process itself" (Greenspan, 1979, p. 18). This has considerable implication, particularly in the realm of identifying the relationship between mental representations produced in drawings and developmental levels of defense and cognition. Noy (1979) addresses the issue also and offers further support for Holt's proposition. This will be discussed in more detail later in this chapter.

The many views on the development of human relationships are beyond the scope of this material, but, insofar as these relationships have considerable influence on the development of mental representations and figurative imagery, some brief points will be noted. Greenspan (1979) describes five stages: (1) *autistic*: undifferentiated self from others; (2) *symbiotic patterns*: differentiated, but still merging; (3) *post-symbiotic*: beginning of the establishment of boundaries; (4) *triangular patterns*: movement from a two-person to a three-person system; (5) *resolution*: leads to an increased awareness of a complex world. Greenspan stresses the importance of the fourth stage and resolution in the fifth stage in terms of this process being essential for the child to move from the pre-operational stage of cognitive development to concrete operational. He places the fifth stage around five to seven years, consistent with Piaget's stage theory. Greenspan describes adult "emotional intelligence" as an adaptation which reflects an interconnected system in which the individual has available prior experiences and is capable of integrating them in a way that makes sense. This allows the individual to function and meet the needs of self and society in the present and future (1979).

In pointing out the similarities and differences between Piagetian and psychoanalytic theories, Greenspan (1979) states that psychoanalysis views "intelligent behavior as one aspect of adaptation" (p. 118), whereas Piaget views intelligent behavior as adaptation. Greenspan also suggests that the process of accommodation of structures should not be viewed as "identical with conscious adaptation," and that awareness is not essential for adaptation to occur. This is important for those who study children's drawings, which frequently communicate processes about which there is no conscious awareness.

Greenspan posits an "internal and external boundary" of the ego and relates internal boundary variables to psychoanalytic theory and external to Piagetian theory. This construct is critical to his presentation for a general model of optimal intelligence and is noted here because the concept of these boundaries is consistent with the idea of unconscious and conscious motivation of behavior. Defense mechanisms, along with the drives, affects, human relations, and superego, are an internal boundary variable, and, when development of defenses is at an advanced stage, they provide protection of the ego without interfering with ego functions (1979). Throughout his work, Greenspan stresses the importance of these two boundaries in that they both influence the process of adaptation and intelligent behavior. In addition to the absence of conscious awareness in some areas of adaptation, Greenspan acknowledges that development defined by internal boundary variables may exist at levels very different from that defined by external boundary levels (i.e. an individual could be functioning at a psychosexual level that is not consistent with his/her stage of cognitive functioning). Regardless of this inconsistency, he believes there is a relationship between these two aspects of development. This, too, is of particular importance to the study of children's drawings where both emotional and cognitive elements are present in all graphic images. In spontaneous drawing, the degree to which either emotional or cognitive elements may be more predominant is indicative of many things: age, genetic endowment, cultural influences and environments, with specific emphasis on the interactions between the child and his environment in the early years. For example, if during the sensorimotor period the processes of attachment and separation–individuation go well, normal cognitive development will follow through the concrete operational stage; if attachment is made, but not satisfactory separation and individuation, representational thinking will be impaired. A mature and flexible ego is necessary for an individual to be able to deal with strong and opposite feelings, like love and hate, and to avoid the regressive process of splitting off bad and good objects (Greenspan, 1979).

A mature, flexible ego is contingent, among other things, upon the kinds of defenses it employs, and-it is this aspect of Greenspan's work that is the basis for this writer's presentation. The interface between cognitive and emotional development is reflected in the content of cognitive function (Greenspan), and, likewise, the content of graphic images is an important element in deciding their relationship and intrapsychic determinants. To summarize Greenspan in his own words, his theory is based on a "conception of a hierarchy of equilibrium states, which at the highest level permit the assimilation of a large number of complex variables into a whole self-regulating system" (1979, p. 295). In his book, Greenspan outlines a schematic level of learning and substages of learning, as he conceptualizes them, and discusses the adaptive capacities and maladaptive patterns for each stage. This provides an excellent review of the material that precedes it, and the reader is referred to this section for a complete, outlined summary of his theory (pp. 380-387).

Noy (1979), mentioned above in conjunction with Dabrowski's work, proposes a theory of cognitive development also based on psychoanalytic psychology. In his opinion, normal mature cognitive functioning must be rooted in a "sound balance between primary and secondary process operations" (p. 170). He describes primary process as "self-centered," but "neither inferior nor superior to secondary process," which is oriented to reality (p. 170). The difference between them is based on modes of organization, a position he supports by citing neurophysiology studies on lateralization (Galin, 1974), which focuses on right-hemisphere mode (i.e. non-verbal representation) versus the left-hemisphere mode (i.e. verbal representation). For example, non-verbal representation emanating from the right-hemisphere mode is rooted in visual thinking and symbolic derivatives of primary process, whereas verbal representation reflects logical, organized, non-visual, secondary process thinking. Noy emphasizes the role of imagery in mental representation which is consistent with that of dynamically oriented art therapists. The "primary process mode is confined to self-related images" which in some form are related to "needs, wishes or past emotional experiences" (p. 173). Noy connects this relation to dream work, which uses condensation, displacement and reversal, and describes the image as a projection of a "seemingly new creation of the inner screen" (p. 173). Adaptation is achieved when an individual can modify himself to meet "changing reality requirements" in his environment, using primary process organization, and can modify reality to meet his own needs, using secondary process organization. Emotional and intuitive responses reflect primary process; logical reasoning indicates secondary process. The cooperation of primary and secondary processes "ensures synthesis of self-interests" concomitant with reality in order for optimal adaptation to occur (Noy, 1979, p. 198).

Various defense mechanisms, the most important of which is isolation, support the function of secondary process as an autonomous thought system. In Noy's view, isolation serves to keep the individual from understanding the "language" of the primary process. He considers isolation unnatural, and that it is the result of educational and societal pressures which produce a separation of primary process operation from logical thinking in the growing child. Therefore, part of the primary process is repressed, and Noy calls this the "language of the unconscious"; part is reflected in conscious expressions of "daydreams, fantasies, contemplation and artistic creation" and becomes a "private language" (1979). In order to compensate for defensive needs and the demands of the environment, which Noy perceives as alien to human nature, man must seek activities that transcend this isolation and synthesize "his primary and secondary process operations" into one act "that is acceptable in society" (1979, p. 212). Like Greenspan, Noy is very clear that both emotional and cognitive development interact and motivate behavior, and to understand human development both must be considered simultaneously.

Developmental Sequences in Children's Drawings: Emotional and Cognitive Factors

Psychologists who have been stimulated by their clinical experience and/or sensitivity to the value of drawings as an indicator of mental process and emotional states have developed many varied tests to examine these issues. Machover (1949) designed the drawing of the human figure test and based much of her work on that done by Goodenough (1926, 1928). Goodenough's work was originally designed for IQ purposes, whereas Machover developed hers as a clinical tool for personality analysis. In the course of administering the Goodenough's Draw-a-Man test, she found that individual drawings often provided rich clinical material that was separate from the intellectual level of the subject. She observed that children scoring the same for mental age would frequently draw very different objects and figures. She also realized that drawings provided an opportunity for the expression of private fantasies, anxieties, and fears, and it became apparent to her that verbal patterns are symbolically "less direct and more subject to conscious manipulation than graphic projection" (Machover, 1949, p. 21). Subsequently, she extended her technique to include adults in evaluating patients in her clinical setting. Her technique has been utilized by psychologists and art therapists, who have found it extremely useful in assessing both mental process and psychosexual development (Levick, Donnelly and Snyder, 1979).

Koppitz (1968) uses only a single drawing of the human figure in her tests because she does not believe a second drawing provides sufficient information to warrant the time it takes to produce. Her analysis of the single drawing is based on thirty developmental items and various emotional indicators. The items are grouped in four categories at each level: "expected," "common," "not unusual," and "exceptional." Validation of the emotional indicators was concluded from the results of a study with seventy-six pairs of children. The conclusions are of particular importance to those working in clinical settings, where therapists are often confronted with the need to distinguish between functional and organic retardation. Drawings frequently reveal mental processes and emotional states operating simultaneously on different levels within an individual. However, little empirical research is reported in this area (Levick, et al., 1979).

Normal sequences of development of children's drawings and the data most referred to by current researchers (Kellogg and O'Dell, 1967; Kellogg, 1969) indicate that all children up to age five, regardless of cultural or ethnic origins, follow a specific pattern. They begin with the scribble, move to shapes within shapes, which become circles, squares, rectangles, and triangles. These in turn become the basis for recognizable images such as animals, people, suns, houses, trees, and other objects. Kellogg's work is an expansion of earlier researchers (i.e. Machover and Koppitz, Buck and Hammer). She has been criticized for not being scientific, but has nevertheless presented considerable data to demonstrate the sequences of the development of children's drawings. Knowledge of these sequences is particularly useful to art therapists in evaluating progressive levels of development and levels of emotional states in regressed, mentally disturbed patients (Levick et al., 1979). A review of these sequences follows.

At about age two, children begin to scribble and discover the look and feel of lines on paper (see Figures 1A and B). There are approximately twenty basic scribbles produced by children, consisting of vertical, horizontal, diagonal circular, curving, and waving lines. They may also include dots. This is a spontaneous expression, but nevertheless seems to indicate that even the very young child has a sense of "figure-ground relationship" (Kellogg and O'Dell, 1967). Kellogg analyzed over one million drawings made by children from the United States and thirty other countries over a period of twenty years. Within this population, she identified seventeen major placement patterns. These will not be listed here, but they suggest that these spontaneous scribbles, produced in the same manner by all children, are the roots of all graphic art. There is no plan for an image or a design in the mind of the two-year-old, and only when it is finished, and then only if the child is asked, is he likely to name it.

The next sequence is the discovery of shapes within the scribbles (see Figs. 2A & B). This usually occurs around age three and is evident when the child begins to make outlines of forms within the scribbles. Some of these forms cannot be classified, but others such as the circle and the square are familiar to the observing adult and not yet known to the child (Kellogg and O'Dell, 1967). Further exploration leads to combining shapes, putting one inside another, adding crosses, etc., initially for the pure pleasure it produces (see Fig. 3). Children tend to produce shapes that have a balanced relationship, and this sequence, which extends to about five years of age, demonstrates more surety and strength in placement of lines and shapes and the development of individual styles. Images are now produced with a plan in mind, and children will readily offer an explanation or story about their drawings. Until children reach the age of about five, there is little difference between the drawings of boys and girls (Kellogg and O'Dell, 1967).

The mandala, usually described as a circle with a cross in it, emerges spontaneously during this period. The mastery of this form leads to the ability to "draw suns, radials and, eventually human figures" (p. 55) (see Fig. 4). Though ages may vary, sequences do not. Only when the above order has occurred do figures appear in

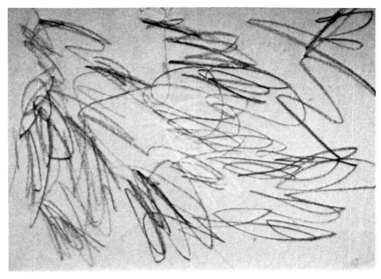

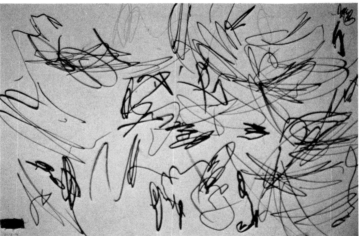

Figures 1A & B. Holly and Doug, both two years old, produced these two spontaneous scribbles, which are typical for this developmental period.

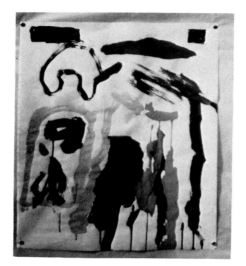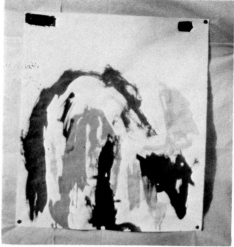

Figures 2A & B. Indira and Gamal, both three years old, appropriately create bright watercolor images of shapes within shapes.

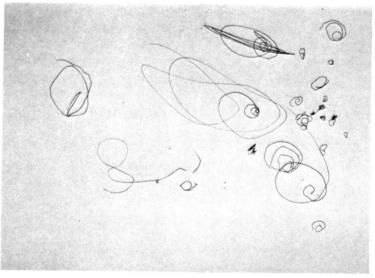

Figure 3. Holly, three years old, is beginning to combine shapes and develop a sense of "figure-ground relationship."

children's drawings. For most children, this takes place around four years of age. The now familiar sun becomes a face; rays are identified as "arms, legs, ears, hair, and head decoration" (see Fig. 5). At first, arms are attached to heads, and markings, regardless of placement, serve more to create balance than realistic representation. According to Kellogg, there is a great concern about balance and this is evidenced in a preoccupation with detail around the head, resulting in "amazing ears and lots of hair, but particularly . . . hats, . . . in every form and size . . ." (1967) (see Fig. 6).

The pictorial stage, which follows the appearance of the figure, usually takes place between the ages of four and five years. Shapes and lines are attached to the "head" and identified as a variety of animals; trees at first look like "an armless human"; the "sun," which by now has become familiar, is combined with other familiar shapes to create a flower. The first crude representations of such objects as boats, cars and houses are the culmination of images emerging from designs, which initially are simple combinations of the different shapes that have been mastered (see Fig. 7). On their own, when they are ready, children will begin to produce pictures from the stories they have heard, their fantasies, their environment. This is true of children all over the world (Kellogg and O'Dell, 1967).

The first pictorial work contains the elements of design in that it may include an image of one object or many images of the same object. Gradually, the child's pictures begin to suggest a story. According to Kellogg and O'Dell, this begins to occur between the ages of five and seven years (see Fig. 8). By this time, the child's dexterity and coordination have increased naturally, and skill in handling various art media also increases. It seems as if there has been a sudden advancement in ability to draw or paint, but for the most part this is due to normal physical development. Kellogg notes a common misconception relating to the stick figure. She points out that this "is not a spontaneous product of child art" (p. 87), but rather something that children, after the age of five, learn from adults or other children who have learned to do this image as a representation of people. Until about twelve years ago, I observed that most children continued to produce the stick figure until they were nine or ten years of age. I refer not only to patients in clinical settings but to children in urban and suburban schools. There appeared to be a comfort in producing this stick figure, totally devoid of sexual

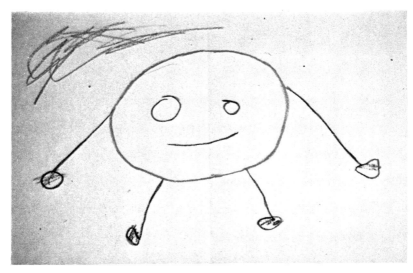

Figure 4. Scott, four years old, has mastered the ability to draw the mandala and connect circles and lines to create a face-like image.

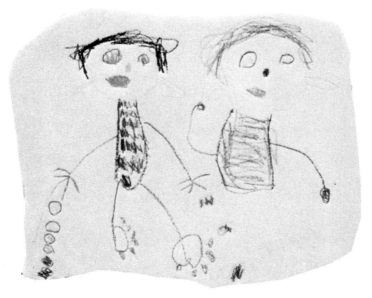

Figure 5. Scott, five years old, combines mastery of lines, shapes within shapes and even the early scribble to produce a recognizable human figure.

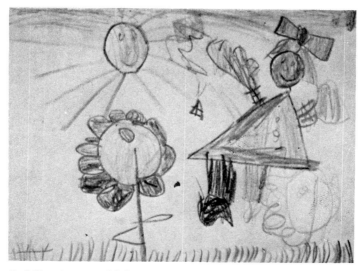

Figure 6. Lilly, six years old, in age-appropriate preoccupation with detail around the head, creates a colorful figure with vivid crayons.

characteristics, that seemed consistent with developmental issues of this period — psychoanalytically speaking, the concept of a moratorium on psychosexual fantasies. During the last decade, this figure representation has been conspicuously absent from the drawings of children observed in these same settings. Nothing was found in the literature to explain this, but the feeling of this author is that television has played an important role in making children more conscious of sexual differences at a much earlier age than reported in the past. This may very well be shortening the latency period.

Kellogg and O'Dell (1967) did not describe children's drawings beyond the age of seven, but, in her later work, Kellogg extended her investigations to include those eight years of age (1969). She writes briefly about anatomical representation of sexual differences in figure drawings and reports that in her studies (at that time), while awareness of these differences is certainly present, "they are certainly not encouraged, if permitted, to portray the bodily signs of sex, except for hair length" (1969, p. 171). Breasts do not appear in drawings frequently and then not until approximately the age of eight.

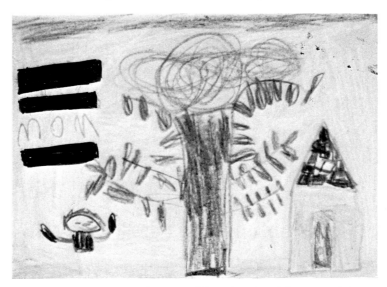

Figure 7. Scott, six years old, has moved into the pictorial stage and draws age-appropriate representations of a house, tree and person.

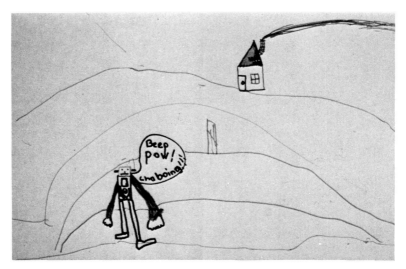

Figure 8. Scott, seven years old, shows greater skill and coordination, which reflects normal physical development, and is manifested in a greater ability to draw and paint.

Other representations that might appear involve the phallus and pregnancy, and generally these schemas are learned from others (Kellogg, 1969). Perhaps television has also lessened the restrictions Kellogg describes.

DiLeo (1973) sees psychosexual orientation reflected in the human figure drawing increasing as the child matures. An early indication is hair length, while differences in clothing appear later. Pre-teen and adolescent girls will pay special attention to eyes and ornaments and begin to illustrate differences in body contour. Boys of this age may draw figures carrying "guns, cigarettes, or other objects to which sexual symbolism is attached" (p. 57). DiLeo also suggests that "intelligent, perceptive sophisticates will portray sex differences at an earlier age" (p. 57). Though DiLeo states it differently than this author, he does seem to support the notion that the child who is exposed to sexual differences at an early age will illustrate them in drawings at an earlier age.

Relationship Between Cognitive Development and Artistic Skill

Hardiman and Zernick (1980) considered the relationship between the structuralist theory of cognitive development outlined by Piaget and the artistic development of children's drawings. They identify stages as a way of describing and organizing "the cognitive strategies children bring to the act of drawing" (p. 12). They cite Piaget (1969), who reports that advanced functional skill results from successful completion of earlier stages, and Arnheim (1954) and Lowenfeld (1957), who support stage theory in terms of understanding artistic growth. Knowledge of this relationship can provide a way for art educators to account for cognitive differences. In western cultures, the relationship between age norms and stages correlates fairly closely; a variation in age, range and stage is evident across non-western cultures. They state that, according to Piaget, the same developmental sequence occurs for all children. Hardiman and Zernick propose no definitive answers regarding sequential stages in artistic growth, and their results do not reflect any select group observed over a period of time. However, they do believe that a definable period in a child's life is characterized by "mode or pattern of behavior" that explains the concept of a stage and its role in development. They list three assumptions that are inherent in the cognitive structure of any stage: (1) concepts in cognitive structures would interact with other abilities; (2) these concepts would be qualitatively different from previous stages; (3) acquisition of functional maturity in the child, for a concept would be the attainment of an adult function as an adult would progress no further. These assumptions also apply to the development of artistic behaviors, with the exception of a "quantitative difference within" as well as "qualitative differences between" stages (Hardiman and Zernick, 1980, p. 17).

Using Piaget's concept of schema, i.e. "schema is one way of observing qualitative change in the behavior of an individual that reflects a class of similar actions that are highly interrelated" (p. 17), the authors make a comparative interpretation between Piaget's concept of schema and Lowenfeld's. It is their assumption that for Piaget, schema equals the behaviors it characterizes, while for Lowenfeld the spatial or figural orientations in drawing represent a schema. For both, a schema implies a process of assimilation has occurred producing a new cognitive structure which in turn leads to a new cognitive organization (Hardiman and Zernick, 1980). A qualitative difference can be understood by comparing "the random placement of shapes in space" in the pre-schematic stage with the "definite spatial order found in the dawning realism stage" as described by Lowenfeld. An example of a quantitative difference is evidenced in comparing the figural schemas in pre-schematic and schematic drawings (Lowenfeld, in Hardiman and Zernick, 1980, p. 17). Both Piaget and Lowenfeld view stage development as "invariant," and that more advanced stages demonstrate new cognitive skills not observable in previous stages, while at the same time still demonstrating those from previous stages. For some time "after a child has left a particular stage of development," quantitative differences may continue to be observed in the refinement of representational drawings, skill in various media, etc. Hardiman and Zernick see as a central problem in studying the development of drawing the transformation and organization of cognitive structures. For transformation and organization to occur, external influences appear to be required in order to make the cognitive structures visible. They suggest that one means for studying the child's cognitive structures is through the understanding of objects drawn by children, which they view as "a surrogate for a mental structure at some particular point." They conclude that the external influence is only part of the explanation for children's cognitive structures; the internal influence is equally important. This concurs with Greenspan's construct of an internal and external boundary.

DiLeo (1973) believes that the realism of young children is intellectual, not visual. He writes, "Young children draw what they know, not what they see" (p. 27). He cites Piaget and Inhelder, who identify two stages in the evolution of imagery. These two stages are static and "imaginal anticipation." DiLeo believes "a bright child might arrive at the second stage at a younger age period; the important point is the succession. Static, then anticipatory, the ages are subject to individual variation." He too stresses that drawings reflect more than intellectual maturity, and much of his work is focused on the drawings as a diagnostic aid for emotionally disabled and physically handicapped children.

Arnheim (1954/1974) extends the intellectualistic theory (noted by DiLeo above) to include the notion that to children things are what they look like, sound like, move like, and smell like. He considers perception a part of primary process, which starts with generalities. Drawings by children of about the ages of three and one-half to four are concerned with generalities, which he identifies as simple, overall structural features. He also believes that artwork proceeds from simpler to more complex images as a result of internal as well as external factors. As the organism matures internally, it is capable of more differentiated functioning. The external world stimulates utilization of this developmental capacity and provides a "variety of directional relations" (p. 188).

Arnheim purports that cognition includes perception, and "visual perception is visual thinking" (1954/1974, p. 14). Perception, which he views as a function of the senses, derives from the biological need for survival and therefore is "purposive and selective." From his perspective, it would seem that perceptions play an important role in shaping adaptive and maladaptive defenses, and, although this is not a subject he addresses at length, what references he does make will be discussed in the following chapter, along with examples of children's drawings. According to Arnheim, images take three forms that fulfill three functions: pictures, symbols and signs. An example of a sign would be a letter, which does not provide obvious visual characteristics of that which it signifies. Pictures reflect "lower level of abstractions" which record "relevant qualities" such as shape, color and movement. A symbol portrays an object at a higher level of abstraction than it actually is (1954/1974, p. 137).

Arnheim (1969) elaborated on his original concept of the relationship between visual perception and visual thinking, and that art education should be a guide to clarification of subject matter and visual representation. Insofar as "thinking calls for images and images contain thoughts" (p. 14), selecting and determining visual concepts involve a process of problem solving which he describes as the "intelligence of perception" (p. 257). He presumes that these solutions are different for each child, and that the making of images provides a means to create some sense of the world. Pictures are not concerned with the outer world alone, but also contain elements of individual experience. The invisible, inaccessible and fantasied are made visible through art expression. "Selection and organization" are necessary to depict or express something (Arnheim, 1969, p. 254).

Gardner, mentioned earlier in this chapter, has for some time been concerned with the relation between drawing and development, and in his most recent work (1980) reiterates what others have stated, i.e. "drawing should not be considered apart from the rest of the child's evolving capacities" (p. 14). He believes that those who have had strong interests in children's drawings have generally ignored the links between these drawings and the rest of the child's "burgeoning powers." As an example, he describes the six-year-old "artist" as a participant in "symbolic play in other areas" and, from this perspective, describes drawing "as part of the overall developmental process" (Gardner, 1980, p. 12). A broad, encompassing study, it is beyond the scope of this presentation. It is mentioned because he raises many questions pertaining to current attitudes toward the teaching of art, and his strong emphasis on the role of drawing in the whole developmental process is consistent with art therapy theory. Gardner pursues the achievement of artistic skills and their relationship to other developmental tasks. This author believes that the image produced by the child can provide invaluable information on dynamic aspects of cognitive and psychosexual development.

Development of Language and Relationship to Visual Imagery

Many researchers have examined the relationship between verbal processes and imagery, and a few of the studies will be cited here. It is not unusual for an art psychotherapist to question whether to be concerned with the graphic productions of an individual who can communicate verbally. The fact is that the two forms of communication often represent parts of a whole. Therefore, two divergent views in terms of their importance to the subject of this work will be presented.

According to Piaget (in Rosen, 1978), speech is egocentric until about the age of seven years. The child speaks primarily to himself and is not concerned with the views of others, nor motivated to speak with others. There are three classes of egocentric speech: the first is repetition (echolalia), which is for pleasure; the second, monologue, is like thinking aloud; the third, dual or collective monologue is where the "other person serves as a stimulus in each child's verbal production." There is no continuity of theme, and others' interests are neither important nor considered (Rosen, 1978, p. 189). The shift from egocentric spech to socialized speech (adaptive communication) is stimulated by a desire to be understood by peers. There are five types: adapted information in which the content relates appropriately to someone else's words, criticism, commands, requests and threats. Language serves as a mediator in interpersonal behavior as cognitive skills increase with age (Rosen, 1978).

Vygotsky (1934/1962 in Rosen, 1978) does not believe that egocentric speech "diminishes gradually in favor of socialized speech" (p. 195). He believes all speech originates out of a social need and splits into "egocentric and communicative speech," both being social but with different objectives. He considers egocentric speech a process by which an individual finds a resolution to some problem. Vygotsky did a study in which he demonstrated that when an older child is frustrated or meets with some obstacle the use of egocentric speech doubles in comparison with either the results reported earlier by Piaget or "natural observations of Vygotsky's subjects." In his view, egocentric speech is internalized and becomes "inner speech," which is retained in adulthood, and remains intelligible and functional for the individual. Vygotsky's work is of particular interest here because some of his data are based on drawing tasks and indicate that the final drawing in a series of drawings (in one case cited by Rosen) reflected an adaptive resolution directed by an expression of inner/egocentric speech (1978). His studies also have important bearing on drawings produced by psychotic patients and the relationship of those drawings to the disturbed speech patterns of this population.

According to Vygotsky, utterances and speech, which he describes as "self-guided," though aimed at communicating to others are initially undifferentiated. When the distinction finally occurs developmentally, egocentric speech goes "underground" and becomes "inner speech" (Rosen, 1978, p. 197). Rosen reports that research supports the findings of both Piaget and Vygotsky and concludes that "adaptive communication in a social context, as observed by Piaget, is not an innate ability" (p. 197). He also points out that the role of socio-environmental factors is an important one in the development of effective interpersonal communication and cites the work of Glucksburg, Krauss and Higgins (1975).

Also relevant to the relationship of language and visual images is the work done by Forisha (1975). She designed a study to extend the findings of Divesta, Ingersoll and Sunshine (1971), who investigated the relationship of imagery to verbal processes. Where the latter used college students as subjects, Forisha's population was children with a mean chronological age of eight years, eight months. Her studies supported the theories of Piaget (1971) and Paivio (1971), which claimed that verbal and imaginal processes are "independent traits whose development parallels each other rather than imagery being the predecessor to verbal as stated by Bruner." However, some interpretations of her data also support Bruner's (1956) views that primitive imagery declines with age and the importance of language skills increases "across all age levels" (Forisha, 1975; in an unpublished paper, Levick, 1979).

Another study by Paivio (in Segal, 1971) indicates these verbal skills to some extent are free from situational context and images. He reports there are no conclusive data supporting his theory, but Haber (in Segal, 1971) offers some support. Haber states "the perceiver may see the world before he knows it . . . at the early stage of processing he does not know what he sees. Thus in the beginning there is the image even before the word" (p. 47).

Summary

The introduction to this chapter identified a fundamental difference between the theories of Sigmund Freud and Piaget. Sigmund Freud viewed the oral, anal and phallic phases as sequences that often overlap. Piaget defines structured stages, each one having distinct characteristics. An example of this would be the "systematic and well-integrated network of logical structures" ascribed to the concrete operational stage "in contrast to the preoperational period which is unsystematic."

A sketch of Piagetian theory was presented, with a brief description of the four major developmental periods: sensorimotor, preoperational, concrete operational, and formal operational. Emphasis was on the first three, which include the age group that represents the focus of this work.

With a view towards integration of these two theories, the work of Dabrowski, Greenspan and Noy was discussed. Dabrowski proposes a theory based on positive disintegration, which he sees as necessary for development, and awareness of inner conflict essential for making choices and decisions which lead to personal growth. Greenspan's work is the most comprehensive, and he examines developmental aspects of Piagetian and psychoanalytic theories. His objective is to evolve a new theory based on both, with a hierarchy of equilibrium states, in which internal and external boundaries are synthesized to an optimum level of intelligent and adaptive function. Noy, also concerned with the interface between cognitive and affective development, suggests a theory of cognitive development based on psychoanalytic psychology. He considers that mature cognitive functioning must be rooted in a balance between primary and secondary process thinking and behavior. To understand human development, according to Noy, it is necessary to consider cognitive and emotional aspects simultaneously.

Dabrowski and Noy address the issue of the role of imagery to a greater degree than Greenspan, but before pursuing this further, developmental sequences of children's drawings were surveyed. The theory most referred to is Kellogg's, who reviewed over one million drawings produced by children from thirty different countries. The most significant fact is that all children draw in the same developmental sequence up to about the age of five regardless of geographic location or ethnic background. Hardiman and Zernick examined the relationship between the Piagetian theory of cognitive development and the artistic development of children's drawings. They believe that knowledge of this relationship can assist art educators in assessing cognitive differences. The role of perception in thinking was considered in a review of the work of Arnheim, who sees thinking and image-making linked and critical in cognitive development. For many, including this author, art is a language, but the relationship between language development and visual imagery must be considered. The work of Vygotsky, Forisha and others in this area was discussed and their results compared to those of Piaget. Of particular importance is Vygotsky's concept of inner speech (an internalization of egocentric speech) as a self-guiding factor in problem-solving processes. Some of his data were obtained through drawing tasks and have important bearing on the adaptive manifestations observable in drawings of normal children and maladaptive indicators in the drawings of emotionally disturbed adults.

Noy integrated artistic, cognitive and affective development in his statement, "Structure of art is based on a combination of primary and secondary process rules of organization, and its perception requires a synthesis of primary and secondary process modes of experiencing and reasoning" (1980, p. 12). The following chapter will examine this synthesis in the drawings of normal children.

The reader is referred to Table I, which will summarize the cognitive, psychosexual and artistic development to the developmental manifestations of defense mechanisms of the ego.

TABLE 1

Correlation of Developmental Lines of Cognitive, Artistic, Psychosexual Sequences and Defense Mechanisms of the Ego Appropriate for Those Periods of Development

Three and Four Years of Age

Cognitive	Artistic	Psychosexual	Defenses
Early Preoperational period	Period of progression from random scribbles to shapes	Anal stage to oedipal stage Issues:	Early Anal
Thinking is centered	Shapes become combined	self assertion	Regression (Incorporation)
Only one aspect of something is attended to at a time	Forms become balanced	control	Reversal
Thought is representational	Beginning of spatial organization	regulate bodily functions	Denial
Symbolization present	Emergence of recognizable objects		Late Anal
Differentiation between self and others present			Avoidance
Animism, realism, artificialism in thought still present			Projection
			Oedipal
			Imitation

Five to Seven Years of Age

Cognitive	Artistic	Psychosexual	Defenses
Animism, realism, artificialism may appear in form of magical thinking	Period of greatest quantitative difference within sequences	Post-oedipal stage	Identification
Early development of logical consistency	Period of greatest qualitative differences between sequences	Major task is process towards resolution of oedipal conflict and identification	Reaction-Formation
	Images reflect movement from a single aspect of an object or form to pictorial sequencing	Positive identification with parent of the same sex	Isolation
			Isolation of affect

TABLE 1 (Continued)

Cognitive	Artistic	Psychosexual	Defenses
Five to Seven Years of Age			
Early development of capacity to understand concepts of classification and conservation	Several objects may be related in one drawing	Negative identification with parent of opposite sex	Simple rationalization
More than one aspect of something can be attended to at the same time	Pictorial images begin to tell stories		Early defenses are available and used appropriately
Seven to Eleven Years			
Concrete operational period	Period of realistic representation of familiar objects	Latency Period	Repression (major defense)
Thinking moves away from centration and irreversability	Relationships are drawn in more orderly fashion	Early Years	Reaction-Formation
Cognitive reversability emerges	Elevated base lines and ground lines appear	Infantile past closed off	Simple Rationalizations
Advancement to a higher stage of equilibrium occurs	Human figures move from static to action related representational images	Parental attitudes and values internalized	Denial
Reasoning can move from the beginning to the end of a process	More frontal and profile views of people and objects appear	Child's attention directed primarily toward learning and peer relationships	Isolation of affect
	Houses and people take on a more proportional relationship	New role models perceived in teachers, movie and television stars and sports heroes	Identification
			Identification with aggressor

Chapter Four

MANIFESTATIONS OF DEFENSE MECHANISMS IN CHILDREN'S DRAWINGS: RELATIONSHIP TO PSYCHOSEXUAL AND COGNITIVE DEVELOPMENTAL ASPECTS IN DRAWINGS

THE review of the literature in the previous chapters strongly supports a developmental hierarchy of defense mechanisms. The authors cited concur that the earliest defenses observed are projection, incorporation, denial and avoidance. These defenses lead to the development and utilization of displacement, repression, reaction formation and rationalization. At the most advanced level, the individual is capable of intellectualization and sublimation. Regression is viewed as a primitive defense mechanism and normal around age three, occurring in combination with other defenses of that period. Anna Freud points out that the child cannot employ projection or introjection until differentiation of self from the outside world occurs. She also suggests that denial, a normal defense in early childhood, is observed through expressions of fantasy, and introjection of the anxiety object may lead to identification with the aggressor. Most authors appear to agree that identification with the aggressor exists at many levels. Anna Freud places reversal, undoing and isolation at an early developmental stage, and the defense mechanisms of imitation, identification and introjection are seen by Anna Freud as specifically related to the onset and resolution of the Oedipal conflict.

The question now arises if in fact these defense mechanisms can be identified in the graphic productions of children. A question raised earlier concerned the relationship of these defenses to normal cognitive development. I propose to demonstrate that knowledge of cognitive and psychosexual development and their manifestations in drawings will lead to identifying defense mechanisms and their adaptive function from a lower to a more advanced stage of development. The following material will be divided into sequences of development with approximate age boundaries; correlations with cognitive and psychosexual stages as described in the previous chapters will be noted. Drawings will be presented and discussed in terms of level of cognitive skill, level of psychosexual development and defense mechanisms. In the previous chapter, some examples were given of early scribbles produced by children under the age of three. This chapter will begin with examples produced by children three years of age.

All the drawings presented throughout this work represent material collected by the author over the past fifteen years. All names have been changed, and specific information about each child has been altered so that confidentiality is maintained. Developmental data were obtained from parents, nursery and elementary school teachers. The population discussed in this section is "normal," and the basis for that classification is that in the pre-school years none of these children demonstrated any extreme abnormal behavioral patterns, and in the school years, all function at an average or better level in their age-appropriate class. Some of the children and their families are known personally to this author; some were met with briefly through professional connections where historical data were also available. Some of the children are not known personally, and their drawings were made available through the professional interest in this study of one of their family members. These facts will be noted with each illustration.

Before proceeding, there are some basic assumptions to be made pertaining to interpretation of drawings and the theory of art therapy presented here. Regardless of training or experience, an art therapist cannot make a valid determination of an individual's cognitive and/or psychosexual development from a single drawing, especially in the absence of direct observation, associations from the artist and/or historical data. However, the well-trained art therapist, knowledgeable in the two domains identified above, can make valid inferences and "educated guesses" that have significance to the field of mental health. Since this is not an experimental study and represents the author's hypothesis, no formal measures of reliability were undertaken. However, the drawings were submitted to former students trained in this method. The results of their evaluation appear in the Appendices. A limited study for validity was also conducted and these results are also included in the Appendices.

These inferences and educated guesses can provide a basis for determining, at that time, if a child's internal and external boundaries (to use Greenspan's terminology) are consistent with each other. Furthermore, this information can determine the need for further evaluation and intervention. This aspect will be elaborated on at length in the conclusion. Regarding defenses, it is the belief of this author that projection and denial are inherent in early scribbles. Where these earliest expressions are reported to be motivated by pleasure, it is this pleasure that is projected onto the paper and is the beginning of what Noy describes as a new creation of the inner screen. Sigmund Freud wrote, "In only a single field of our civilization, art, has the omnipotence of thoughts been retained" (1913, in Rothgeb, 1972, p. 85). The principle of the omnipotence of thought is the same principle which governs magic and the animistic mode of thinking discussed in Chapter Two in relation to the defense of projection. These views support the author's belief that the early scribbles are expressions of internal experiences and projecting them onto paper is an adaptive process.

Concomitant with this is the relationship of denial to fantasy described by Anna Freud. The first scribbles also serve as a form of play that leads to fantasies about forms emerging in the scribbles. The eighteen-month-old to two-year-old child who takes crayon (or any graphic media available) in hand and begins to scribble finds it very difficult naturally to stay within the boundaries of the paper. The author's experience over the years with her own children, grandchildren and other toddlers has demonstrated that initial efforts to restrain the child (who is old enough to understand commands) from going out of those boundaries are totally ignored. It is suggested that this unwillingness to comply reflects the child's denial of awareness of reality. As the child develops, these two defenses are more clearly illustrated. At this level of development, projection and denial are natural mechanisms employed to cope with internal and external stimuli.

For further clarification, the author's criteria for identifying the manifestations of defenses in drawings are included at the end of this chapter. The reader is referred to these criteria when reviewing the illustrations in relation to specific defenses (see Table 2).

Three and Four Years of Age

In cognitive theory, this marks the early phase of the pre-operational period that Piaget places between the ages of two to seven years. Thinking is centered, and only one aspect of something can be attended to at a time. The child now is capable of representational thought and can symbolize objects that are not present. On an interpersonal level the child can differentiate between self and others, but interactions are motivated by physical or egocentric needs (Rosen, 1977).

From the psychoanalytic view, the child of this age is dealing with the tasks of the anal stage and early Oedipal phase of development. Major issues are self-assertion and control, emanating from the external demands to regulate bodily functions. Two defenses employed during this period may be *avoidance* of seemingly unpleasant shapes and smells and *projection* onto objects in the environment of unpleasing qualities and attitudes perceived in their environment. (Anna Freud). These may be observed separately or in conjunction with other primitive defenses mentioned above.

During this period, graphic images progress from random scribbles and shapes to combined shapes, balanced forms, beginning of spatial organization, and emergence of recognizable objects. Arnheim describes this as a time when children begin to depict visual concepts of objects in their environment in a primitive abstract form. Images are normally isolated at this time and are analogous to parallel play. Arnheim points out that the selection of these visual concepts of objects from their environment is part of the process of problem solving, and in this way the child is making order out of disorder.

Illustrations
(All names of defenses will be italicized)

Figure 9 was produced by Holly at age 3. This is the same child who produced Figure 1A mentioned in the previous chapter. Holly is the second child of an art therapist mother and professional father. Holly and her brother (five years her senior) were and are encouraged to draw freely whenever they wish. These drawings by Holly (and her brother, whose work is described elsewhere) were offered as examples for this section by their mother.

After completing the drawing, Holly announced it was "a man with funny hair." Without her identification of the object, one sees the scribble, circle, line, transformed into a primitive representation of a figure. The elements of the image are age appropriate and indicate she mastered the scribble and shapes within shapes sequence. It reflects a *projection* of an image with great attention to detail on top of the head. This in part could represent the concerns at this age with balance (Kellogg), but the subject matter also reflects a need to cope with the perception of some figure in the environment. The preoccupation with the hair is the internalization of a previously mastered achievement (scribble), and the focus on one part is consonant with the cognitive capacity to address only one aspect of an object at a time. However, the intensity with which the (scribbled) hair is executed is *regression* to a more primitive and gratifying expression. This is not unusual for a child of this age who, as Mahler describes, is working through separation–individuation and may still be in the rapprochement phase. Holly's identification of the figure as a man suggests the beginning of Oedipal concerns with daddy.

Indira, whose beautiful painted image of shapes within shapes (see Fig. 2) was shown in the preceding chapter, also produced the pictures shown in Figure 10. This little girl from India was 3.4 years old when we met in a nursery. She was intrigued with colors and in age-appropriate manner used them spontaneously and non-representationally. During one of my earlier visits she had asked me to help her outline her hand on the paper. Within a very few minutes several other children, including the older ones, were all engaged in this task. It is not unusual for three year olds to want to do this over and over; it is a concrete projection of part of the self onto an object in the environment (in this case, the paper) and allows the child to exercise some control over it. Figure 10 was done during a later visit, and as she drew she named some of the forms and permitted me to write the names on her picture, which she then presented to me. The large yellow form is a horse; the turquoise form on the left, a cat; the pencil form at the bottom left, Mr. Uppity, and the orange form to his right, an umbrella. Scribbles are still in evidence, but separated from the representational forms. Cognitively and graphically, she had achieved the capacity to represent the features and, in a primitive way, the ears of the cat. There was no opportunity to pursue

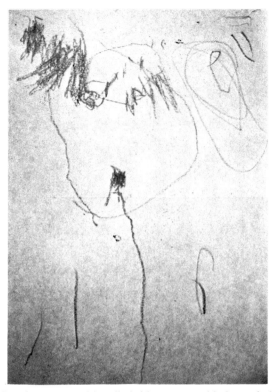

Figure 9. Holly, three years old, called this "a man with funny hair." Images and defenses manifested are age appropriate and include projection and regression.

the origin of the image of Mr. Uppity, but his isolation both in placement and use of a different medium (pencil) from the other forms (magic marker) reflects her use of *isolation* as a defense. This manifestation is obvious with knowledge of her cultural background — a minority in that nursery. It was also known that she was the youngest of five children and infantilized in the home (report from the nursery school teacher).

Knowledge of this data suggests that the nursery school demands and her minority role may have been sources of anxiety which led to the use of this defense. Having the opportunity to observe her in play, I was struck by the extremes in her behavior. As her drawings

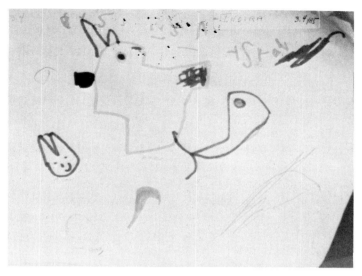

Figure 10. Indira, three years, four months old, uses color spontaneously and non-representationally in age-appropriate manner. Major defense in drawing is isolation seen in isolation of objects and use of pencil for one form as opposed to magic markers for all of the other forms.

indicate, she could function in an age-appropriate manner for a period of time, then suddenly withdraw, isolate herself, or do something she knew would require a member of the nursery staff to separate her from her peers. Indira's need to withdraw herself socially, coupled with the isolation of both an object and an affect (Mr. Uppity produced in a different medium) in a drawing of many objects, supports the notion that this defense may be a major defense for her at this time. Another apparent defense was regression. While regressive behavior is common at this age, she resorted to it to a greater degree than others. That, coupled with the image of Mr. Uppity and the anxiety manifested in the rendering, suggests close observation of this child and communication with the family to make the daily transition from home to school as smooth as possible.

Tony was just three years of age when I was introduced to him at his nursery school. Although the youngest full-time child attending that school, he was one of the most self-sufficient and happiest.

Figure 11 is an example of the many tempera paintings he produced. His handling of the media is very sophisticated for a three year old. Compared to Indira's and Gamal's pictures (see Figs. 2A & B) in Chapter Three, which are age appropriate, he demonstrates a boldness and control not evidenced in their paintings. He was more consciously experimental than they in that he placed one color next to another or over parts of another color form; he did not appear to be controlling the media by isolating one color from another as they did. An interaction we had points to his ability to pictorialize, represent objects realistically and utilize *imitation* at an earlier age than most children. Unfortunately, we have no illustration of his production as the images were executed on a chalkboard, but they will be described. During one visit, he invited me to draw with him, took a small chalkboard and colored chalks for himself, and gave me similar supplies. He proceeded to draw a tree, sun, grass, and clouds and told me to do the same. His use of colors for each symbol was appropriate, but each was rendered in a primitive (but not inappropriate) way. For example, the sun was begun with a crude circle and filled in with yellow chalk in quick scribbled lines; the tree, a series of brown lines for the trunk and green ones for the leaves, and so on. As we worked, he frequently looked at my images and finally commented that mine were different. I asked if he would like to know how I made them different, and he promptly handed me a blank chalkboard and said, "Show me." As I produced each symbol, I explained how to add the rays around the sun, fill in the trunk, make leaves with repeated circular scribbles on top of the trunk, include a ground line and short vertical lines on top of it for grass, and outline clouds. He immediately copied my drawing almost perfectly and was pleased with himself. I also was pleased with him, and I told him so. Knowing the rules of the nursery, he cleaned all the chalkboards and put everything away. I was disappointed that there would be no record of this. Several weeks later on another visit to the nursery I saw him at a table drawing on paper with magic markers. He motioned for me to come and see what he was doing. Tony was reproducing the symbols in the same schema that we had worked on together several weeks before. This child was not only able to *imitate*, but he was also capable of *projecting* mental representations of objects not in his present sphere of perception. He was delighted with these pictures and put them in his folder. His drawings indicate that he was at an advanced level developmentally both cognitively and affectively. His use of symbols, space and organization of these elements into a schema represents a process of assimilation (Piaget and Lowenfeld). The use of *imitation* as an adaptive defense placed him in the Oedipal stage according to Anna Freud. His interest in the tree and the sun, two symbols often identified with father in the literature, suggests his beginning to experience Oedipal concerns around masculine identification.

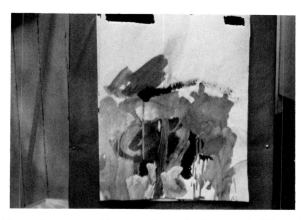

Figure 11. Tony, three years old, uses color and paint more boldly and experimentally than most children his age, suggesting he was advanced in all developmental domains.

The following two examples provide an interesting contrast to the drawings by Tony and Holly. Harry was just four when he produced the pictures shown in Figures 12 A and B within a period of several weeks. Figure 12A shows little evidence of control, little separation of colors, and is for the most part a muddy blob. This is not age appropriate, and questions regarding his development would not be out of order. Figure 12B indicates he was capable of controlling the media and therefore implies Figure 12A is a manifestation of *regression*. The repetitive use of one color and one form speaks of a need to master and control some aspect of his environment. He was very articulate and, sometimes when relating incidents, sounded like "a little old man" (a shared opinion of the nursery school staff). At other times, he would behave extremely immaturely, dependent, and unable to readily accept assistance from someone who was not familiar to him. He was assessed as a very bright child by the nursery school staff, and I agreed with this assessment. His erratic behavior was attributed to the fact that his mother was expecting another child within a few months and he was having difficulty dealing with this. The drawings communicate that he was using *regression* and *avoidance* predominantly and the intensity and pressure necessary to produce the smeary mess in Figure 12A contain elements of aggression and/or angry feelings which have been *displaced* onto the paper. The use of *displacement* was also apparent in his play with the other children and interactions with the staff. In spite of his obvious intelligence, Harry was not coping well with the advent of a sibling, and his drawings mirror those of a child closer to the age of two and one-half to three years rather than one of four.

Leon, 4.1 years of age when he produced Figures 13A and B, was attending a highly structured nursery at the time. He offered no comments about the first drawing but said the second was "a kind of hamster," and this was written on the picture by a member of the staff. Leon seemed to have barely mastered the scribble and shapes-within-shapes sequences, and I was told these were fairly typical of most of his graphic productions. He was an interesting child to observe because, although his movements and speech seemed slow and pressured, he could communicate verbally in an intelligent manner that was age appropriate. I was informed that there was no evidence of any organic impairment, and some of his slowness was attributed to the fact that he had been hospitalized that year for a form of ear surgery. Hospitalization is often traumatic to children, and if there was any prolonged period of illness prior to surgery, it would have significant bearing on their emotional and cognitive development. I present this example because Leon was viewed clinically as average for his age. I consider his drawing to be on a two- to three-year-old level of development, with no evidence of regression, because this level was consistent in his many drawings I saw. There does seem to be some *undoing* in his description of the hamster (i.e. it is not a real one, only a "kind of" one). On a verbal intellectual level, he seemed to be aware this was not an adequate image.

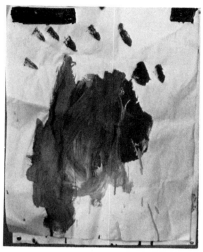

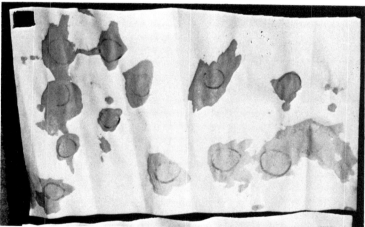

Figures 12A & B. Harry, four years old, produced both paintings within a period of several weeks. The picture on top shows little evidence of control, whereas the picture on the bottom indicates that he is capable of controlling tempera paint. This marked difference in levels of artistic development indicates the use of regression as a major defense and may lead to maladaptive coping styles.

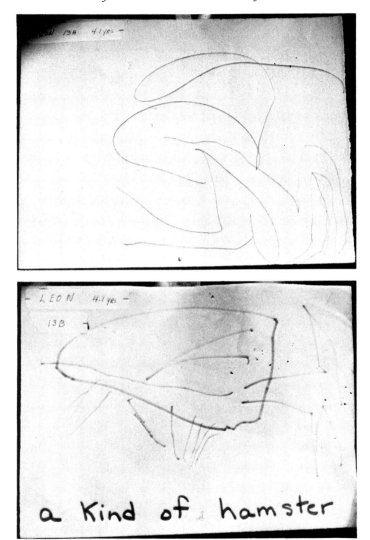

Figures 13A & B. Leon, four years, one month old, did these and similar line drawings repeatedly. They are not age appropriate and indicate that his artistic development is at age two to three years. The immaturity of the images also suggests some concerns about his psychosexual development as well. He directed the writing of the title on the bottom picture, and on an intellectual level he seems aware that this is not an adequate image of a hamster.

Lilly was a little past age four when she drew the pictures shown in Figures 14A and B. She is the daughter of a colleague and was often invited to draw pictures for her father and this author to use in classes for art therapy students. Both pictures beautifully demonstrate all the criteria that identify capacities inherent in this stage of development. She controlled the media, drew mental representations that are recognizable and are understood here as *imitations* of objects perceived in her environment. She was already attempting to attend to more than one aspect of something simultaneously (i.e. the inside and outside of the house) (see Fig. 14A). Consistent with her age, she *denied* and *avoided* reality by placing them side by side. The house (often a symbol for mother) and the sun mentioned above are Oedipal symbols and the curved lamp base and shade are considered feminine forms. At age four, she was faced with Oedipal issues, and her drawings and the defenses depicted suggest no cognitive or emotional problems at the time they were produced. There is an interesting fact about the spontaneous painting of the three figures and it relates to Greenspan's observations of the period. Lilly was the younger of two children, but only represented three figures. According to Greenspan, the triangular relationship between child and parents is singularly important in the process of cognitive adaptation and is equally important in the process of interpersonal relationships. Although not evidenced in the drawing, knowledge of Lilly's sister points to the use of *denial* and *undoing* in the omission of a fourth figure in the painting. All of these things are natural for this age.

Five to Seven Years of Age

Most researchers in cognitive theory tend to mark the end of the pre-operational stage at around six years of age and the beginning of the concrete operational stage at seven years. These arbitrary demarcations do not allow for the rich interaction between the Oedipal (and the post-Oedipal) period of development described in psychoanalytic theory and the transition in cognitive development from pre-operational to concrete operational. This is a critical period in both areas of development.

Cognitively, the child is beginning to develop logical consistency in thinking, and everything he has accomplished prior to this period

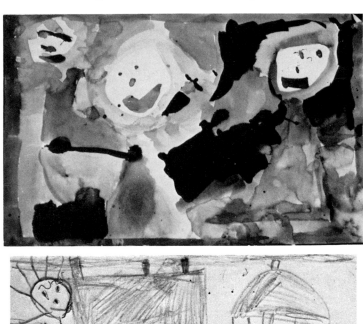

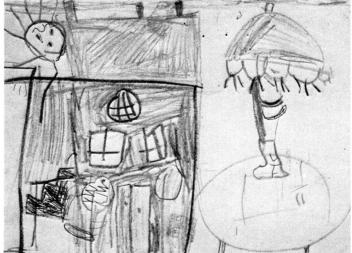

Figures 14A & B. Lily, four years, two months old, demonstrates all criteria that identify capacities inherent in this stage of development in both paintings. Artistically, she is approaching the pictorial stage; on a cognitive level, she can attend to more than one aspect of something at the same time; on a psychosexual level, she is using Oedipal symbols and defenses of denial and avoidance.

is in preparation for a greater capacity for equilibrium. Animism, realism and artificialism, which Piaget connects to egocentrism, may appear during this time in the form of magical thinking. There is a developing capacity for understanding the functions of classification and conservation and the ability to organize and manipulate the environment. Limitations of the pre-operational period begin to disappear. Perceptual clues become less misleading and the child begins to recognize that the way something looks may not necessarily be reality.

As noted briefly above, the triangular relationship, resulting from the Oedipal set, plays an important role in enabling the child to perceive a new system of interactions between more than self and one another, as experienced in the early dyadic relationship. Greenspan believes the degree of successful resolution of the Oedipal conflict will have bearing on the degree of drive influence on concrete operational structures. It is further believed here that this resolution also influences whether defenses become adaptive or maladaptive.

In psychosexual development, a major achievement of this period (defined here as the post-Oedipal) and in the process of resolution of the Oedipal conflict, is identification. In psychoanalytic theory, this is viewed as positive if it is made with the parent of the same sex and negative if made with the parent of the opposite sex. In addition to identification, other major defenses are reaction formation, simple rationalizations, denial, and isolation of affect. This does not mean to say that those defense mechanisms employed earlier are no longer called on. It was stated elsewhere that as the ego matures it has at its disposal a wide variety of adaptive defenses to employ in different situations, and drawings by children of this age should reveal these age-appropriate cognitive and emotional aspects of adaptive ego function.

During this period, the graphic productions of children seem to show the greatest differences, a conclusion derived from clinical experience. The growing child acquires new perceptions of known objects in the environment. The acquisition of new perceptions and intellectual awareness of new objects and people in the environment also develops. These now become internalized. The degree to which this occurs differs for every child without interrupting the sequential pattern of artistic development. It is during this time that quantitative differences within a stage and qualitative differences between stages (Hardiman & Zernick) are most discretely observed. Therefore, some five year olds may still be dealing with one aspect of something and represent it in a drawing singly or repeatedly, while other five year olds may have progressed to the pictorial sequence where their pictures contain several related objects and may even tell a story. During this time, all children are becoming more interested in depicting known objects representationally, and the increased control of media allows for more detail in drawings. Proportions in subject matter will begin to appear but remain simple until more complexities are perceived and understood. As the child approaches seven years of age, there should be some awareness of the base line and horizon line and appropriate placements on paper. The drawing of the human figure will be less static (i.e. begin to show movement), and sex and role differentiation may be evident. The cultural milieu and the process of the Oedipal resolution have considerable input in determining this latter element. The human figure drawing, more than any other image, reflects body image and role identification, and cognitive maturation alone does not insure a healthy self-image.

Color will remain secondary until pressure (from teachers and others) is brought to bear on its relationship to a specific object. There are a number of studies that claim that a specific color signifies rage while another signifies depression, and another happiness, and so on. In two decades of working with thousands of hospitalized patients and school children, little support has been found for these conclusions. For the most part, association to colors (and they have been solicited wherever possible) reveals that color choices in spontaneous drawings are personal and most frequently determined by subject matter, as well as cultural and parental values. The increased application of many different colors in the process of picture-making is concomitant with the natural conscious experimentation prevalent in the child's pursuit of gratification through graphic expression. Further amplification of the concrete operational period and the latency period will be addressed below. For the age group under immediate consideration (5 and 6 years), images of human beings generally are more individualistic than realistic or externalized. Lowenfeld (1939) attributes this to a feeling response and calls these images "haptic." However, Lowenfeld's concept of haptic images does not extend to the productions of inanimate objects where more conventionalized patterns, in which there are no or little expressions of feeling, may prevail (in Alshuler & Hattwick, 1917/1969).

Illustrations

Scott was five years old when he produced the pictures shown in Figures 15A, B and C. For earlier examples of his work the reader is referred to Figures 4, 5, 7, and 8 in Chapter Three. This young, prolific artist is Holly's older brother, and, as reported in discussion of her drawings (see Figure 1 in Chapter 3 and Figure 9 in this chapter), a variety of art media is always available. His illustrations abound with "surrogate" (i.e. substitute) mental representations of an object from some point in time. The reader is reminded that in spontaneous drawings subject matter is individually determined and symbolically manifests latent (unconscious or preconscious) wishes, fears, and fantasies. Cognitively, Scott could attend to more than one thing at a time and told his mother that his picture is a "boy, a girl, and a rainbow" (see Figure 15A). He was dealing with relationships, and each object has individual, realistic features, but the proportions of the objects in relation to each other are unrealistic. In all of these aspects, his work was age appropriate and connotes that he progressed in the pictorial stage. The same holds true for Figure 15B, which he described as a "clown and boy bouncing balls together." Let us examine these two drawings in terms of psychosexual development. We assume Scott was in the Oedipal stage, as defined by psychoanalytic theory, and struggling with forbidden longings for mother while at the same time recognizing, on some level, the need to be like father. There were other complications in this little boy's life. His mother was expecting another child and if his new sibling had not yet arrived, she was expected imminently. The exact state of that situation is not known, but in spite of this lack of information important inferences can be made from his drawings about Scott's adaptive mechanisms. Little boys of five learn about girls from the important women in their environments and about rainbows from stories they have heard or picture books they have read. That these had special meaning for Scott is evident from their inclusion. Further, the projection of these objects, along with the balls (also in

Fig. 4) and the clown, suggests a "dynamic distortion" summoned forth by the tension connected to the original form (Arnheim). Some differentiation between male and female is obviously perceived and depicted in the attention given to the hair and the fuller trunk on the girl, implying a dress. At this age, tension with members of the opposite sex originates with the parents (or caretaking persons), and Scott used *avoidance* to defend against the tension. This is recognizable in the way the clown is leaning away from the other figure and the number of objects between the two figures. In this fashion, he also *reverses* his wish to be close. *Denial* was employed by making the female (mother or sister) the same size as the boy (a *projection* of himself), which also implies he was as big as father and imparts the early use of *identification*. Children's stories tell us rainbows are something special and may even have a pot of gold at their end. This may hold great promise for obtaining all the wonderful things a child could dream of. Scott not only reversed and avoided his unacceptable Oedipal wishes, but was already seeking his rewards outside — the beginning of *sublimation* and *reaction formation*. In Figure 15B, Scott *displaced* all his awe and fear of father (the rival for mother) onto the figure of the clown. After all, clowns do all sorts of tricks — some that are perceived as wonderful and some that are perceived as frightening. At the same time, Scott was portraying *identification* with the aggressor in the projection of the larger, more detailed figure of the clown, for there is part of the artist in all the parts of the picture. In this view, in the former drawing, the image of the girl, whether symbolic of mother, sister or both, could also represent the aggressor — mother for having a new baby and sister for intruding on his space. Figure 15C, drawn in honor of Thanksgiving and labeled "turkey," points to yet another defense. A turkey is not easy to draw at any age, and Scott devoted all his attention and most of the space on the paper to the one subject. His graphic skill was centered on the face of the turkey, and in comparison with his other drawings the figure is reminiscent of scribbling in the body area. In this difficult task, Scott's image reflects an earlier artistic sequence and he regressed graphically, used *isolation of affect*, and indicated that he could utilize, yet contain, his *regression* in an effective manner. These drawings illustrate how one five year old had at his disposal a number of defense mechanisms ranging from the very primitive one of *avoidance* and *denial* to the more advanced consonant with his age and stage of psychosexual development (i.e. *displacement, reaction formation* and *identification*).

Figures 16A, B, C, and D were also produced by Scott, but a year later. At six years of age, while on a family fishing trip, he resorted to a now familiar mode of expression to master and cope with a frustrating experience: Scott did not catch a fish. He titled each picture: (A) "jumping fish"; (B) "fishing girl"; (C) "she caught a fish"; and (D) "she has it on her chane" (his spelling). His relationships of objects are more realistic, and within the span of a year he became aware of the horizon line and could illustrate it appropriately. The excitement of the experience is isolated in the movement of the jumping fish (the only moving image in the picture), thus indicating *isolation of affect* (see Fig. 16B). With knowledge that the artist is a boy, it is apparent he has used *projection* and *displacement* in the portrayal of a girl succeeding where he failed (see Fig. 16B). Even if the facts were not known, these defenses would be inferred through the *reversal* of the (self) image from boy to girl. This is confirmed in the next two drawings in which Scott identified the figures as girls but omitted female characteristics (see Figs. 16C & D). *Reaction formation* is suggested by *displacing* gratification of his wishes onto another. No indication of sex differentiation in the last two figures, an artistic ability Scott demonstrated at age five, is *regression* to an earlier sequence (which would include *denial*) and points to his growing capacity to call on cognitive and emotional resources at a more advanced level than was seen in the scribbled body of the turkey a year before.

The next series of illustrations requires and deserves a more elaborate introduction. The few represented reflect not only extraordinary communication, in terms of cognitive and psychosexual development of the six- to seven-year-old first-graders who produced them, but the sensitivity of their remarkable teacher. The acquisition of these graphic images was fortunate and accidental, the result of a visit to a friend while attending a meeting in a midwestern state. During the visit, our hostess, who teaches first and second grade in the small elementary school of this somewhat isolated but socio-economically and culturally homogeneous community, became intrigued with the discussion regarding the format of the work. Subsequently, she shared her own format for teaching reading. Without any formal knowledge of art, music or movement, she employs all three modalities to impart the relationships of signs and symbols to

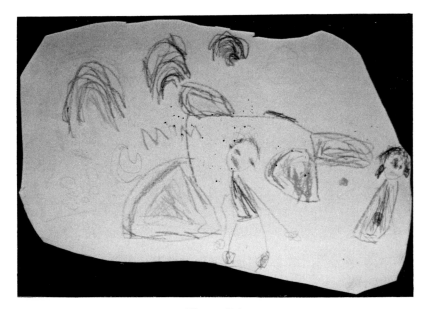

Figure 15A

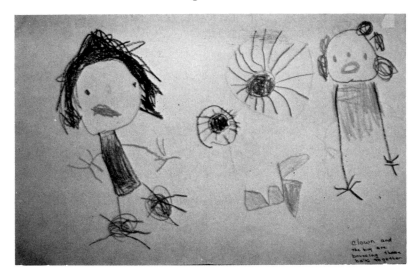

Figure 15B

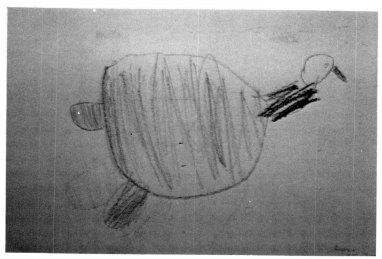

Figures 15A, B, & C. Scott, five years old, did these drawings in colored pencils and called the first one a "boy, a girl and a rainbow"; the second picture he called a "clown and boy bouncing balls together," and the third picture he called a "turkey."

words and their meaning through expressive participation in art, music and bodily movement. While the final product of the children's images is the result of individual spontaneity, personal selection of subject matter and imagination, initially there is a specific structure imposed. The children are provided with an eight-by-ten sheet of paper, pencils and crayons. They are instructed to write eight specific words and to illustrate them on one side of the paper, and to illustrate those on the reverse side first outlining each image in pencil. Together we reviewed the drawings produced by the entire class for one lesson. The inferences and "educated guesses" made from these drawings about the academic performance and emotional status of each child seemed incredible to their teacher, but were obvious to this author, and gratifying in that they correlated with her observations and confirmed her concerns about some of the lower-functioning children.

There are limited psychological resources (predominantly school psychologists who do routinely required IQ tests) and no specialists

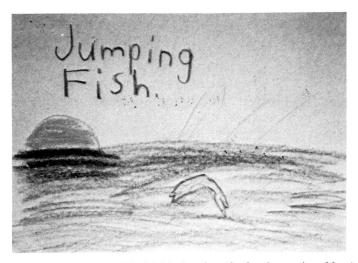

Figure 16A. Scott, six years old, did this drawing (the first in a series of four) after a family fishing trip. He is now aware and capable of illustrating the horizon line — a normal advancement in cognitive and artistic development. Isolation of affect is seen in the movement of the "jumping fish," the only object indicating movement in the picture.

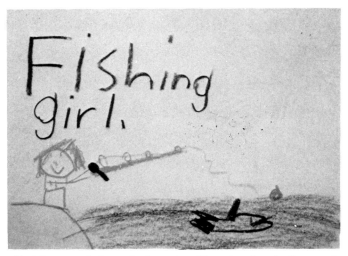

Figure 16B. The second picture in the series of four drawings by Scott at six years of age. Knowing the artist is a boy and capable of distinguishing male and female characteristics, he is manifesting projection and displacement in the portrayal of a girl as the fisherman instead of himself.

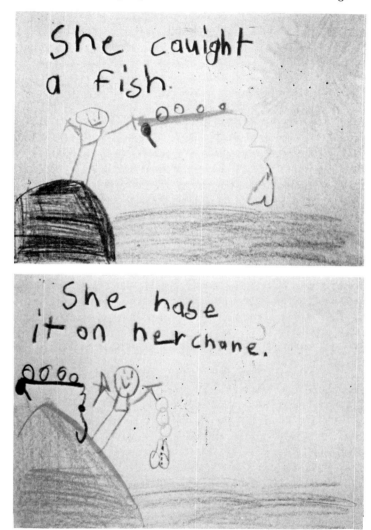

Figures 16C & D. Scott, at six years of age and in the third and fourth drawings of this series, also illustrates the use of reversal as a defense, along with projection and displacement. He identifies the figures as girls but omits any female characteristics. Regression, denial and the beginning of reaction formation are also indicated.

or facilities for children with learning disabilities in this community school. The only way this teacher deals with children who do not seem able to master first-year school work is to have them repeat the year with her. She feels that this added time helps them to gain more security with the basic learning tasks before proceeding to the next level. Considering the circumstances, these children are most fortunate. In many urban communities, unfortunately, it is not uncommon for children to be promoted to advanced levels before they are ready. The wealth of material the teacher made available for this project would provide sufficient data for a separate study. The few examples presented here have been selected for their diversity and richness of projected thought and feeling. Our friend's enthusiasm for this study impelled her to solicit a fourth-grade teacher at her school for drawings from her class. Some of these will be reproduced and discussed in the section on that age group.

In sharp contrast to Scott, Bill, also six years of age, was glaringly inconsistent in his graphic productions (see Figs. 17A & B). His movements fluctuated in revealing cognitive and psychosexual developmental indices. His examples for "killers," "sleep," "strip" on the one side (see Fig. 17A), and for "Iran" on the other (see Fig. 17B), manifested age appropriateness intellectually, emotionally and artistically. The other images look as though they were done by a much younger child. The forms were isolated by virtue of the assignment, but *isolation of affect* is still observable in separated spots of color in certain forms (i.e. the orange face illustrating "cry" and the orange face and green balls drawn for "kick"). *Regression* was his major defense and can be seen in the extensive return to scribbling and drawing of shapes within shapes, which are expressions normal in the late oral and anal stages of development. His Oedipal concerns emerged in the figure drawings. The images for "killers" and "Iran" strongly suggest *projection* (of hostility) and *identification with the aggressor*; "strip" shows a fusion of male and female characteristics (breast and phallus are both present); and the stick figures were a *denial* of any sexual identity.

Lewis (6 years old), on the other hand, maintained the same level of functioning throughout. He created an image that is appropriately related to each word, all executed in a manner that placed him in the pictorial sequence (see Figs. 18A & B). There is some *isolation of affect* in the omission of any evidence of a person connected to the

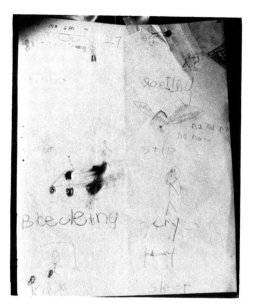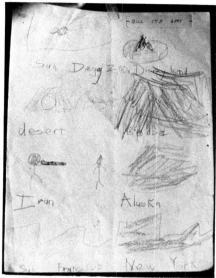

Figures 17A & B. Bill, six years old, graphically represents inconsistency in his developmental lines. Some of the images are age appropriate, while others appear to be drawn by a much younger child. Regression is his major defense and is seen in the repeated use of scribbling and shapes within shapes.

symbol of the gun for "shoot," and a great deal of feeling is attached to this symbol vis-à-vis the strong use of color. *Avoidance* is exhibited in the side view of the nude figure for "strip," unusual in that a profile view is representative of an advanced level not commonly encountered in a six-year-old child. Overall, Lewis's images attest to his ability to synthesize outer and inner stimuli and defend against provocative thoughts without interference in appropriate performance for his age. His steady externalization of mental representations also points to an apparent capacity to *sublimate*, thus obtaining gratification for some instinctual wishes through an accepted form of expression. This is certainly true of Scott, also.

Renee, age six-and-one-half years, is an interesting child. She handled the media well, and her images display symbolic relationships to the words they are illustrating (see Figs. 19A & B). Her drawings raise the question as to whether she is still in the pre-operational stage, dealing with only one aspect of an idea, or moving

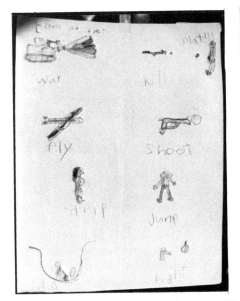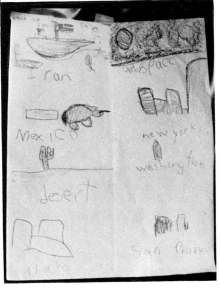

Figures 18A & B. Lewis, six years old, is in the pictorial stage artistically and reflects cognitive development consistent with his age. Defenses illustrated indicate he has an appropriate number of defenses available and uses them well to cope with natural Oedipal issues.

into concrete operations and demonstrating a more advanced capacity to form a symbolic abstraction of an idea. For example, she drew only the head for "cry" and "sing" and made it explicit. In the drawings for "jump" and "run," there appear to be distortions of the legs that could suggest a concern for balance. It is more likely a serious attempt to portray the identified activity, hampered by her lack of skill. We conclude from her overall graphic representations that Renee was performing at the late pre-operational stage and, from her representation of the more complex image "circus," that she was beginning to show evidence of movement into the concrete operational stage. Generally, she focused on one view to illustrate the word. She manifested the defense mechanism of *isolation of affect* by coloring in only certain parts of figures for the words "jump" and "talk." In addition to this defense, the consistent omission of body parts on all the figures is seen as an expression of *denial*. Artistically, this child was perfectly capable of drawing a complete figure, yet the only one that comes close to being complete is the upside-down figure on the elephant. The art psychotherapist must consider omissions in drawings as unconscious slips of the crayon. Renee was communicating her normal developmental cóncerns around the body — concerns arising from Oedipal conflict. Her figures are the dynamic distortions that Arnheim describes and as such are projections of her anxiety about her self-image. Identity was in process, not yet resolved, and characteristics of male and female were not clearly differentiated. Her illustration of "zoo" — the legless bear behind bars leaning out toward the bird on the bar in space — was a lovely expression of this post-Oedipal child trying to "break out" and spread her wings and exemplified the beginning of sublimation. Without Renee's associations it can only be conjectured that, insofar as both the bear and the bird are representations of herself, she inhibited that part of herself that the bear represents by putting it partially behind bars reaching out to the bird, which symbolizes the freedom to fly in the environment.

Jon, also six-and-one-half years of age, drew the image in Figure 20 repeatedly, in a variety of media, so that it was almost like a doodle. This young artist is the son of a colleague, and when this was drawn, Jon was exhibiting no behavior problems and considered by his first-grade teacher to be very bright. His picture is a castle, an imitation and condensation of many such castle pictures in children's books. The drawing points to the same conclusions as those derived from Renee's drawings. The figures in the lower archways are on a much more primitive level than the castle structure, and Jon's preoccupation with the "triangular relationship" is marked by the two sets of three windows, the three archways and three figures. His lingering tie to the dyadic relationship is symbolized by the two turrets, one on each side of the top of the castle. Jon's major defenses at this time were *isolation of affect* (no color in the figures) and *denial* of body parts, in addition to *imitation* and elements of *sublimation*. Imitation is reflected in his attempt to copy someone else's rendition of a castle and, like Renee (see Figure 19B), he inhibits parts of the self by placing some figures behind bars and draws other parts of self as freestanding figures in the archways.

The following examples were produced by several seven year olds and are presented in this section because they also exemplify the transitional aspects considered inherent in this period.

Eva drew the pictures shown in Figures 21A and B within a short

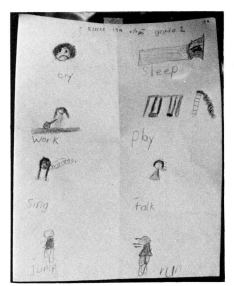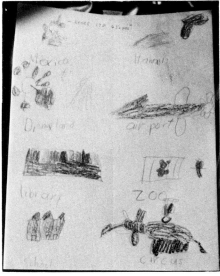

Figures 19A & B. Renee, six years, five months old, handles the media well and shows indications that she can function in all developmental domains on an age-appropriate level. Inconsistent representations of figures and male and female characteristics not clearly defined suggest she is struggling with normal developmental concerns around body image. Major defenses depicted are denial and isolation of affect.

time of each other and visually elucidated the gamut of feelings flooding the Oedipal child. In both figures, Eva demonstrated she had achieved cognitive skills that enabled her to attend to more than one aspect of an object simultaneously and even produce complex pictorial images (see Fig. 21B). She was aware of the horizon line, and her organization and spatial relationships place her well into the concrete operational stage (see Fig. 21A). Eva was very conscious of her sexual identity, but *denied* it in Figure 21A. One cannot tell if the rider is male or female, yet we know she was capable of detailing characteristics vis-à-vis the highly skilled representation of the horse. *Isolation of affect* is seen in the contrast between the bright sun and dark picture, and *denial* is manifested in the asexual figure and the indiscernible object on the right side of the picture. It looks like a hurdle, which is a fitting symbol for the task of identification. Fig-

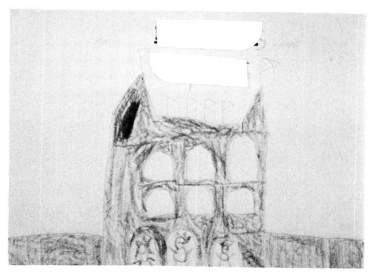

Figure 20. Jon, six years, five months old, drew this image over and over, suggesting the need to master its symbolic meaning. The castle is on a higher developmental level than the figures drawn in the archways and point to his normal concerns related to the Oedipal period. Defenses illustrated are isolation of affect, denial, and imitation.

ure 21B is rich with projected images and mental representations of things perceived as good and bad. "Pandora's box" contains Eva's symbols for blindness, cold feeling, germs, death, etc., as well as a good spirit. The images of the monster and the good spirit are somewhat less mature than the figure of Pandora (a projection of Eva's self-image), which is replete with flowing black hair and elaborate dress. All the fantasies and fears experienced by children during this period are exquisitely and symbolically portrayed and, at the same time, defended against in the sublimated expression of a familiar myth. She *displaced* all of her fantasies, fears and wishes onto Pandora, but the picture of this mythological character (and Eva) is undaunted. She stands upright and looms larger and more realistic than any other image. It seems that Eva knew that identification carries with it the pressure of applying controls that are awesome, but identification was imminent. This is supported by the fact that both parents are professionals and hold responsible positions.

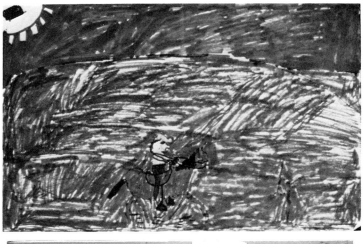

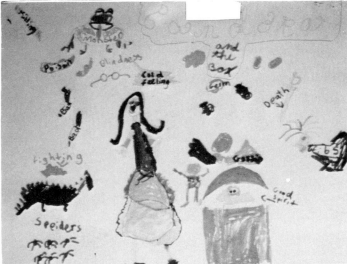

Figures 21A & B. Eva, seven years old, did these two drawings within a short period of each other. Cognitively, she is in the concrete operational stage and artistically can create complex pictorial pictures. She titled the bottom picture "Pandora and the Box" and in both pictures vividly portrays ideas and feelings flooding the Oedipal child. Defenses reflected are denial, isolation of affect, and displacement.

David, age seven years and in the first-grade class discussed previously, drew the pictures shown in Figures 22A and B. Cognitively, psychosexually and artistically, he was on the same level as Eva. He was more explicit in his ambivalence regarding the process of identification and incorporated both male and female characteristics in the illustration for "strip" (see Fig. 22A). On both Figures 22A and B he expressed the utilization of *denial* through the absence of any sexual characteristics elsewhere and *avoidance* through (higher level) drawings of side views of figures. *Isolation of affect* is implied in the visual mental representation of "screem" (his spelling) and the colorless face on the colored figure in the illustration for "play."

Allen, the same age and another member of this class, was very dexterous and did an excellent job of rendering Mickey Mouse to illustrate "Disneyland" (see Figs. 23A & B). The absence of realistic figures is glaring, and his *denial* of sexuality predominates in the nine symbolic representations of a figure.

Yale's drawings are included because, in addition to the defenses used by the other children in this sample, he also employed *regression* to cope with anxiety emanating from the process of identification and projected onto his graphic images of figures (see Figs. 24 A & B). Where appropriate control of the media and relationship within a single object and between others prevails in Figure 24B, Figure 24A shows much less control and a return to scribbled areas to make a form. Yale also utilized *undoing* where he covered over his stick figures with crayon. It should be remembered that instructions from the teacher stated only that each image was to be drawn in pencil first. The use of color was the decision of the child. In this particular series, most of the children, when they did draw a stick figure, seemed content to leave the pencil image unembellished. Yale's pressured covering over of the line figures mirrors dissatisfaction with the initial conceptualization, repeatedly doing and *undoing* it.

In the Introduction, this period was stressed as critical for cognitive and psychosexual development. Drawings produced during this transitional time are an invaluable source of information and literally draw the path from imitation to identification in pursuit of the Oedipal resolution. These drawings also communicate a considerable amount of data regarding the repertoire of defense mechanisms available to cope in an adaptive fashion appropriate for

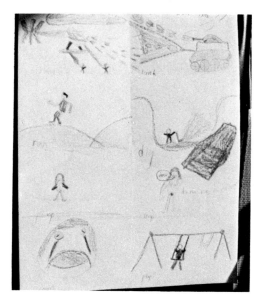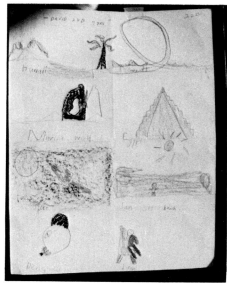

Figures 22A & B. David, seven years old, reveals cognitively, artistically and psychosexually that he is experiencing all of the thoughts, feelings and concerns related to this stage of development and coping well. Defenses illustrated are denial, avoidance and isolation of affect.

this age. It is also believed and well supported in the literature that adaptation in the psychosexual sphere at this time leads to greater freedom for intellectual accomplishments in the ensuing years.

Seven to Eleven Years of Age

The years from seven to eleven are described by Piaget as the *concrete operational stage*. In psychoanalytic theory it is called the *latency period*. As stated in several places previously, all children of the same age do not achieve the same level of functioning at the same time. This does not necessarily signify an impairment of cognitive development or emotional disturbance, only that each child moves through these sequences at his own pace. The emergence of advanced levels of performance in intellectual and graphic representations will be reviewed briefly along with the psychoanalytic perspective of this period. The illustrations will cover ages eight through ten years of age and will be presented sequentially in order to demonstrate some

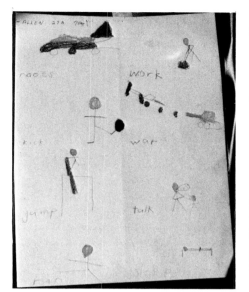 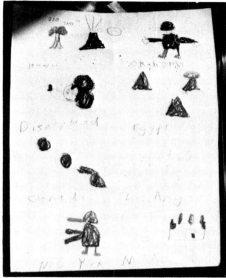

Figures 23A & B. Allen, seven years old, shows great dexterity in handling the art media and is consistently age appropriate in all domains. His major defense in these two pictures — denial — is seen in the overt omission of realistic figures.

individual differences.

According to Piagetian theory, this expanse of middle childhood heralds a movement away from centration and irreversibility and advancement to a higher stage of equilibrium. The child can now reverse procedures and carry out an operation in both directions. Reasoning can now be applied to a process from the beginning to the end of that process. Circles and squares can be identified and differentiated from each other even though both are closed forms; straight lines can be recognized as different from curved lines. All thought processes are becoming more consistently logical and are carried out internally, whereas in the previous stage internal cognitive actions were sporadic and equated with intuitions (Piaget, in Rosen).

Latency, spanning approximately the same years accorded to the concrete operational stage, is a time when "the infantile past is closed off . . . and covered with amnesia" (Anna Freud, 1965, p. 35). Psychoanalysts traditionally view it as a sexually quiescent time.

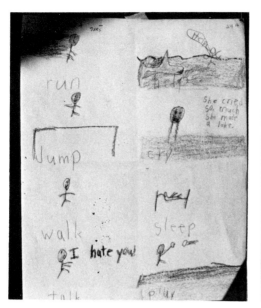
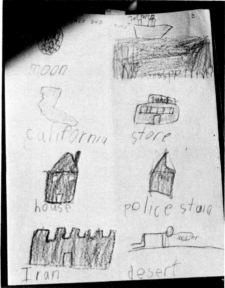

Figures 24A & B. Yale, seven years old, gives evidence that he can function cognitively and artistically on an age-appropriate level in the picture shown on the right, but shows much less control in the picture shown on the left and manifests more primitive defenses of regression and undoing.

Greenspan questions if this is so, and drawings by children at this age observed over recent years seem to indicate that there is a greater freedom in the expression of material with a sexual connotation than previously noted. It was also suggested above that the reason for this may be due in part to greater exposure through television and a change in sexual mores. Nevertheless, most investigators concur that the latency child's attention is directed primarily towards learning, peer relationships and new role models perceived in teachers, television, movie and sports heroes. Parental values and attitudes are internalized and the superego is the psychoanalytic structure conceptualized as the controlling force to keep thoughts and actions within acceptable boundaries dictated by the environment. The major defense employed here is repression, which is the basis for the adaptive or maladaptive employment of other defenses the child has at his/her disposal. Greenspan lists reaction formation, simple rationalizations, denial, and isolation of affect as other appropriate defenses for this level of development. Identification, especially with the aggressor, must also be included along with intro-jection. Reversal, generally connected to the late anal or early Oedipal periods of development, according to Greenspan will also occur here. He correlates this defense to Piaget's concept of cognitive reversibility and as an example describes how some feelings of hate for a person may be reversed by some feelings of love. On an un-conscious level, this is the dynamic underlying reaction formation. Anna Freud reports that this latter defense is understood only when it is observed in the process of breaking down. However, graphic ex-amples have been presented previously that did manifest this defense in the developmental process, and illustrations that follow will amplify this further.

Artistic development is immersed in the realistic representation of familiar objects, and their more orderly relationships are achieved through the increased use of elevated base lines and ground lines (Hardiman & Zernick). In spite of the pressure placed on children, particularly in the school system, to become proficient in verbal ex-pressions of their experiences, fortunately some children continue to draw at home and in school. For many children, this pressure closes the door on the appreciation of fine art and art as an expressive mode. For other children, for whom art may be an important means of expression, this bias may lead to their isolation. Human figures may remain static in the early years of this period, but later become more representational of active movements and frontal and profile views. Where houses and people may have been the same size in the pre-operational stage, they take on a more proportional relationship.

Clinical observation over the years has shown that children dur-ing this period focus on those things that are of paramount interest within their peer group and project them into their drawings. Ex-amples of this will be noted in the following illustrations.

Illustrations

Criteria for age-appropriate manifestations in drawings for the pre-operational stage and this stage have been defined at several places herein. To avoid burdening the reader with their repetition in conjunction with each illustration, it will be assumed that these criteria are evident unless otherwise noted. Attention will be focused on defense mechanisms and how they are manifested.

Ned, eight years of age, was performing satisfactorily in his second-grade class. However, his drawings indicate that he was still in the transitional period between pre-operational and concrete operational stages, and Oedipal and latency stages (see Figs. 25A & B). Like Yale in Figures 24A and B, but not quite to the same degree, he used *undoing* as a way of coping with the anxiety around body image. His stick figures are all colored over. There is some evidence of *regression* in the illustrations for "jump, "Hawaii," "moon" and "fire station." Their lack of control in the use of color, scribbles to fill in space, and primitive shapes within shapes are in sharp contrast to the much more mature images for "Iran," "New York" and "laugh." *Isolation of affect* is apparent in all of the drawings in Figure 25A vis-à-vis isolated spots of color (feelings) in all of the images. Ned's presentation for "fight" is an interesting example of *reversal* and the beginning of *reaction formation*. It is difficult to imagine that this child could intellectually and graphically conceptualize two figures fighting, particularly in light of skills demonstrated throughout his sixteen images. Yet, he drew two tiny heads, reversed the anticipated angry expression associated with the word "fight," and put smiles on the two faces. If not completely repressed, angry and obviously unacceptable feelings were being suppressed and their opposite displayed. This is consistent with the process of *reaction formations*. *Denial* of sexual identity is inherent in the use of the stick figure as a representation of the human form, and even when Ned drew a full figure (New York), he chose to omit the entire bottom half of that figure.

The next example raises some interesting questions in terms of the overuse of specific defenses and the bearing this has on the development of a mature, flexible ego. Carl was eight years old and, according to his teacher, was exhibiting no major problems in keeping up with his second-grade school work. He was capable of comprehending his assignment and conceptualizing and visually representing an appropriate symbol for each word and place. He chose not to use color, and every image is executed in pencil with many erasures, suggesting insecurity and anxiety about his performance (see Figs. 26A & B). This also reflects a poor self-image, borne out in the primitive, incomplete images of the figures. They are drawn on a five-year-old level and inconsistent with the more mature renderings

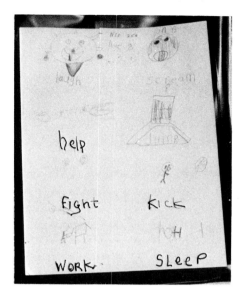 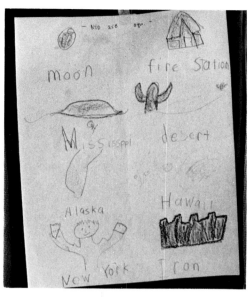

Figures 25A & B. Ned, eight years old, pictorially indicates he is in transition between the pre-operational and concrete operational stages, and Oedipal and latency stages. Defenses illustrated are undoing, regression, isolation of affect, and reversal.

for "laugh," "frown," "desert," and "Iran." To confuse the issue further, Carl drew side-views clearly, a capability that is age appropriate. Carl communicated through his subject matter that he understood and could respond adequately to demands requiring thought processes. He was having considerable difficulty resolving issues around identification. The defenses used here are *denial* (absence of body parts), *undoing* (absence of any color/feeling), and *avoidance* (profiles), all of which originate during the anal stage of psychosexual development. It would seem that because of the different levels of the graphic images, *regression* as a defense should be included. There is a sense in this case that these immature figure drawings represent the degree to which Carl mastered this sequence in his artistic development rather than a regression to an earlier stage. His intellectual capacity enabled him to draw on a higher level where the resolution of the task does not provoke so much anxiety. The rigid, limited use of earlier defenses at this time would be sufficient reason to investigate this child's behavior patterns outside of

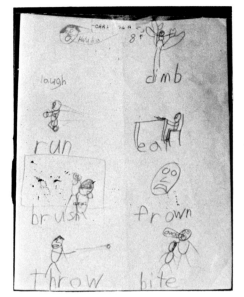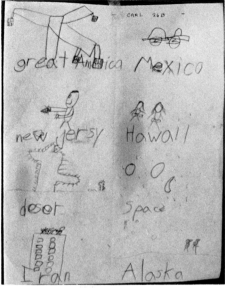

Figures 26A & B. Carl, eight years old, appears cognitively to be able to carry out the assigned task, but his images reflect insecurity, anxiety and poor self-image in the primitive, incomplete figures and which are drawn on a five-year-old level. Artistic and psychosexual development, at this point in time, are delayed in comparison to his cognitive development, which appears age appropriate.

the classroom. There is legitimate concern, supported by the literature, that if this limited repertoire of presently adaptive defenses is not expanded, Carl will experience difficulty in adolescence when the normal psychological upheaval of that period is upon him.

Nina, also eight years old, appeared to be functioning well and appropriately in all domains (see Figs. 27A & B). Her major adaptive defense was *identification*; all of the stick figures have some color added to them for the purpose of differentiating sex roles (six figures in Fig. 27A). There is some evidence of *denial* of sexuality in the use of the stick figures for the human form, but this is expected at this period and suggests that *repression* of the Oedipal conflict is active. It is also not a rigid mode of expression; two figures are more realistic ("Texas" and "play"). Filled-in areas are reminiscent of scribbles but are contained within outlined boundaries and connote a limited and appropriate use of *regression*. *Isolation of affect* is manifested in some of the pencil-outlined forms juxtaposed to colored forms on Figure 27B.

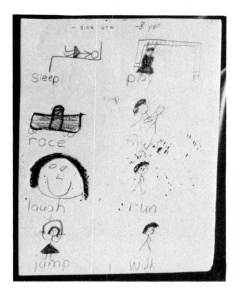 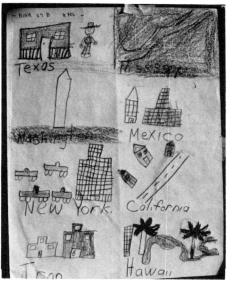

Figures 27A & B. Nina, eight years old, is functioning well in all domains. The major adaptive defense illustrated is identification, and there is some evidence that repression is operative. Also depicted is the controlled use of regression, denial, and isolation of affect.

However, the overall presentation of Nina's images points to the productive employment of a number of defenses for different situations.

Ron, the same age as Nina and in the same class, had no difficulty representing males and females and made a further distinction in the activities he ascribed to each sex (i.e. kicking and running for male figures, and Hula dancing for the female form) (see Figs. 28A & B). *Identification* is clearly present, as well as *isolation of affect* and *regression*. The second is apparent in the consistent omission of color in the face of every human and animal form. This symbolic representation of the separation of thought from feeling is natural at this time and leads to the inference that *repression* is effective. The reader may be inclined to believe that some of Ron's images reflect a looseness or "style" of drawing. Ron's style of drawing is certainly different, for example, from Nina's, but style should not be confused with inconsistency in graphic representations. More will be said about this in the concluding chapter, but it is addressed here to highlight the examples of *regression* in Ron's drawings. This seemed to be an important defense for him and was brought into use when there was some sense of insecurity, observed in the projected image which is less mature than others. Sharp examples of this are images for "bark," and "zoo," and "school" (see Figs. 28A & B). Why these words caused some anxiety, which was then projected into a "dynamic distortion" of an object, cannot be determined without his associations. Given his school record, there seems to be no reason for concern, but should the use of regression increase and become a rigid method of coping with stress, further exploration should be considered.

Another example of the importance of differentiating between style and inconsistency is exemplified in Figure 29. This was drawn by Scott, who by now should be well known to the reader, when he was eight years old, two years after the picture shown in Figure 16 was produced. In the interim he continued to employ art materials to master and work through problems, using realistic and symbolic images. This drawing was unlike anything Scott usually did. Dynamically, he was struggling for control and achieved it to a great degree by *regressing* back to shapes within shapes and, with great pressures of the crayon on the paper, repeatedly doing and *undoing* and redoing each shape. Because of its totally different structure from all of his other pictures, it is not "just a design." There is information that sheds some light on events immediately preceding this drawing. In discussing the picture with Scott's mother (who is a colleague), she recalled two incidents that occurred almost simultaneously prior to Scott's going to his room and immersing himself in the drawing. His father had left on a business trip that would keep him out of town for several days, and "immediately after he was told that a good friend was separated from his family" (his mother's words). It is believed Scott's picture was a way of trying to "undo" the fear of father not returning and losing his father as had his friend. Scott's resources were many, and this is an excellent example of his maturing ego and an artistic expression of how it functions.

The influence of a particular art medium on the final product was noted in the previous chapter on art therapy. When a medium is difficult to handle, the manner in which it is used can be telling in terms of motoric and cognitive skills as well as artistic development. Randy, nine years of age, chose watercolor and produced the pictures

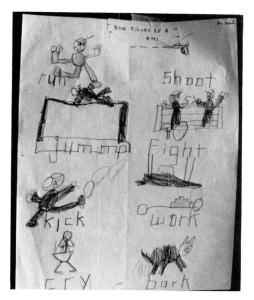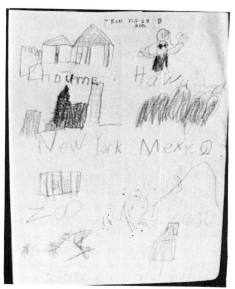

Figures 28A & B. Ron, eight years old, clearly distinguishes between male and female characteristics and activities ascribed to each sex. The major defense manifested is identification, and images infer repression is effective. Ability to function in all three domains is parallel and appropriate for his age.

shown on the Frontispiece on thin white paper. This is no simple accomplishment. Even though he also used magic markers to draw in lines, his images attest to his well-advanced capabilities. Randy is the youngest of three children, and his mother is a professional artist. Like Scott, he has easy access to art materials and spends many free hours drawing and painting. These four examples were all done spontaneously within a short time of each other, and projections of different thoughts and feelings are externalized through each creation. The images in the Frontispiece make a clear differentiation between male and female and document the availability of *identification* as a defense. Two of the images in the Frontispiece suggest sadness and happiness, respectively. *Isolation* and *denial* are represented in both (denial in the absence of body parts). These pictures together show the two extremes of an affect. Randy had *introjected* external values, internalized the conclusion that sadness is not acceptable, and put the symbol for this feeling behind bars. In contrast, the happy faces have broken through the bars and imply the beginning of

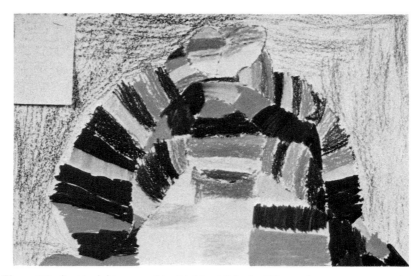

Figure 29. Scott, eight years old, did this strikingly different image as compared to previous examples (see Figs. 15 & 16) in response to an anxiety-provoking situation. In an effort to control and master anxiety, he regressed to a more primitive level of drawing using shapes within shapes and illustrated the defense of undoing.

reaction formation. A fourth image in the Frontispiece looks like a sailboat and is typical of subject matter drawn by boys of this age in his particular community. However, his sailboat is floating in space, and he *denies* its ability to move (and, symbolically, his own mobility) by omitting water and someone to sail it. This inference is made because Randy's other images communicate his skill in drawing and knowledge of ground lines. Greenspan (1979) writes that the ability to make "simple rationalizations" begins in the concrete operational stage. He believes that when the child describes feelings in terms of degrees (e.g. more or less, or not as good as), that child is beginning to rationalize. Certainly, Randy made such a distinction between the sad figure and the happy faces. It seems he was communicating that sadness can be present, but not in the "whole figure," and only if it is contained (symbolically behind bars). Conversely, happy faces are not contained, but Randy suggested by omitting the bodies that just because "he" was smiling it does not mean he was "completely" happy. From this perspective, he may indeed be representing rationizations about some of his own ambivalent feelings about certain issues. While this is highly suggestive from his pictures, associations from Randy would be necessary to validate whether this was a conscious manifestation of different feelings (rationalizations) or an unconscious expression of an unwanted feeling (reaction formation). Overall, this young boy's ability to symbolize, *displace* and condense in image-making mirrors his growing capacity to sublimate.

The next two drawings are presented because they exquisitely point out the power of the image and how in certain situations it provides much more data than clinical observations do (see Figs. 30A & B). Our original intent was to include these two examples in the next chapter, which discusses graphic images manifesting psychopathology. The fact is that Lori, age ten when these were produced, was described as an above-average student in school and having no problems in any other area, and the decision was made to include her drawings here. At that time, her parents were having marital counseling, and the therapist's supervisor, addressing another sibling's problem, suggested an interdisciplinary family evaluation. The parents were committed to therapy and agreed to bring in their children for a verbal interview, an art therapy family evaluation, and a movement therapy assessment of the family notated during the other two sessions. They also granted permission for the entire process to be filmed (Nagy, Levick & Dulicai, 1978). The direction given to Lori for Figure 30A was to draw "anything she wanted to" and for Figure 30B to "draw a picture of her family." Eighteen-by-twelve-inch paper, crayons and magic markers were provided. The conceptualization, organization and spatial relationships all relate an age-appropriate representation for cognitive and artistic development. The consistent and predominant use of such immature defenses as *regression, denial, reversal* and *undoing* defined psychosexual development at a much lower level. The form in Figure 30B indicates that Lori was capable of cognitively and artistically representing a complete figure on an age-appropriate level. Therefore, the pervasive scribbling over of images which are drawn on a much lower level indicates the use of regression. An attempt at *identification* appears in Figure 30B but is *reversed* by the symbolic projection of self in the trash bag and the omission of some family members (requested in the initial directions). She denied the stress at home and called her image "the house of happiness." This also suggests an effort on Lori's part to use *reaction formation*. She further filled in areas with primitive scribbling, *undoing* some of the first forms. The subject matter and associations validated that this child, under great stress, had little access to her intellectual resources and had to call on defense mechanisms consolidated normally at age two to four years. Prior to the interview, the parents reported that Lori knew very little about their personal problems and was in no way affected by the troubled marital relationship. The evaluation demonstrated otherwise, and the consultant agreed that her graphic images, plus a disturbing movement pattern in her interactions with parents and art therapist, revealed her inability to cope with the situation even before it became evident in manifest behavior.

It was reported previously that the fourth-grade teacher (in the south midwest school discussed) asked her students to create some drawings for this presentation. She suggested that they draw anything they wanted, as well as a picture of their families. Paper, pencils and crayons were provided. The exact age of each child was not given, only that they were all between the ages of nine and ten years and functioning at an average or better-than-average level in classroom activities. Three examples have been selected to demonstrate how children of about the same age express themselves differently in graphic images, but incorporate the same defenses on an age-appropriate level. Dianne's cognitive and artistic development is well documented in her free picture of Snow White and the Seven Dwarfs and her family drawing (see Figs. 31A & B)). Romantic fairy tales are a typical subject for pre-adolescent girls, and Dianne's anxiety about emerging sexual fantasies is suspected by the consistent use of *isolation of affect* (no color) and *denial* (omission of the dwarfs' bodies and feet on all of the figures) in both drawings. Role differentiation is unquestionable, and *identification* is positive and an effective defense. In the family picture, Dianne drew a little girl with the same hairstyle as Snow White (her fantasied self-image) within the outline of her mother's lower body.

Herb (see Figs. 32A & B) and Don (see Figs. 33A & B) were both concerned with acts of aggression and appear to have used *displacement* to externalize their own aggressive feelings and *project* them onto fantasied graphic representations. Don drew unrealistic, pumpkin-head figures in his image of someone being stabbed (see Fig. 33A), an image on a lower level than his obvious drawing ability, seen in the heads of the family members, would lead us to expect (see Fig. 33B).

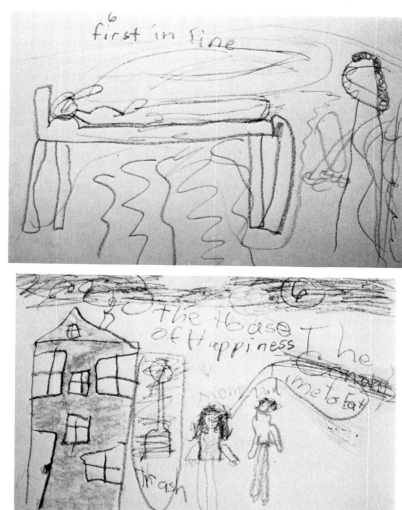

Figures 30A & B. Lori, ten years old, did these drawings "first in line" and "the House of Happiness" during a family evaluation and revealed that psychosexually she was functioning on a much lower level than she was on cognitive and artistic levels. She consistently manifests the use of immature defenses of regression, denial, reversal, and undoing, and efforts to use identification are incomplete.

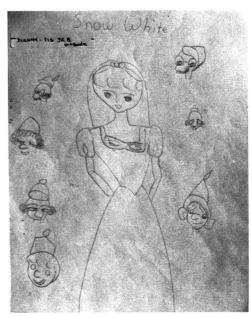

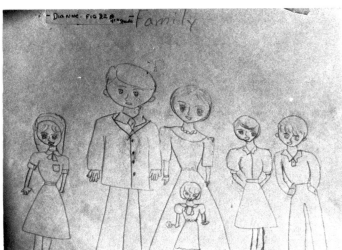

Figures 31A & B. Dianne, ten years old, is representative of a typical pre-adolescent who is illustrating her fantasies through images of romantic fairy tales and manifesting appropriate defenses of isolation of affect, denial and identification to cope with normal anxieties of this period.

Herb's shooting scene reminds one of ships and things from outer space. Both boys used *isolation of affect, denial* and had the capacity to *sublimate.* Their drawings imply that they had not only *identified* with the male figure in their environment during the Oedipal period but that they may also have *identified with the* (perceived) *aggressor.* Don seems to have experienced more concerns around this issue and manifested it by omitting all body parts below the head in the family picture and *regression* in the less mature rendering of the human figure in Figure 33A. It should be pointed out that even though Herb drew complete figures for the family, his constricted use of space is as much an expression of *denial* as Don's omission of the bodies.

Summary

Insofar as this chapter has dealt exclusively with examples of the manifestations of cognitive, artistic and psychosexual developmental aspects and defense mechanisms in children's drawings, it seems only fitting that this material should be summarized graphically. The drawings of five children were made available to this author through different sources. The drawings will be presented sequentially for each of these children to demonstrate their progression through some developmental sequences and the developmental expansion and utilization of defense mechanisms as part of their ego function. Information about the children will be provided only as it pertains to the subject of this work and offers validation for inferences, but will be disguised to maintain confidentiality. Three of the children are from one family and not known to us. Their mother, a student in the field of education, learned that this work was in progress and offered her children's drawings; the other two are the children of a family member known since birth to this author.

Elysa is the oldest of four children and was born in the late sixties. Figure 34A was done when she was eight-and-one-half years old, B when she nine-and-one-half years old, and C when she was ten years old. In the first two, developmental aspects overlap. She was able to represent complete figures and objects and was aware of ground lines, but she separated sky from ground like a younger child. The relationships between objects were both appropriate and inappropriate. Defenses were *isolation* (single figure), *identification,*

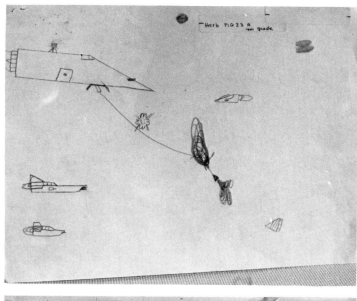

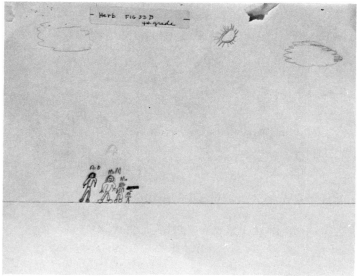

Figures 32A & B. Herb, ten years old, reflects normal concerns at this age with acts of aggression and copes with them by externalizing, projecting, and displacing these feelings onto graphic images. Identification and identification with the aggressor are adaptive defenses illustrated.

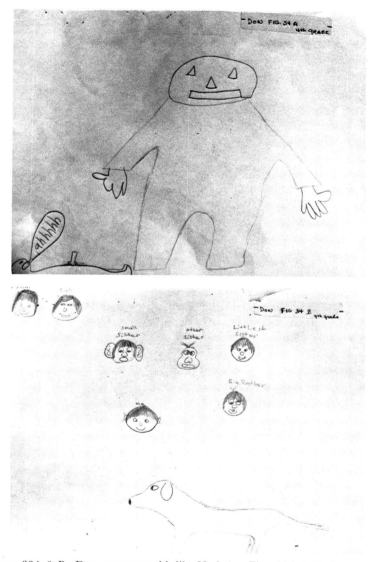

Figures 33A & B. Don, ten years old, like Herb (see Figs. 32A & B), is expressing similar normal concerns related to aggression. Unlike Herb, though, he appears to have more concerns and manifests the primitive defense regression along with those identified in Herb's drawings.

avoidance (profile), and (controlled) *regression* (scribbled hair and sky). Her pictorial representations reflect earlier acquisitions of *imitation* and *projection*. Figure 34C is a highly *intellectualized* design. I do not know if this was an assignment that limited the use of colors. Even so, her final product is a study in *doing* and *undoing* (forms are completed, then divided into several parts) and *isolation of affect*. Her ability to execute such a complex image speaks to her advanced level of thought processes and artistic development. More information is necessary regarding the degree to which this was a spontaneous picture before inferring other defenses. Figure 34D, a drawing of a human figure, is more than adequate in the representation of cognitive and artistic development for a ten year old. While the image reflects a great deal of sophistication, it also reflects anxiety around body image. At age eight-and-one-half years, Elysa very definitely drew a little girl. At ten, she appeared to be having difficulty defining whether the figure is a male or female. The figure could be either, but it seems that the person is wearing an earring. Concerns of definition are natural for the pre-adolescent, and she dealt with them by utilizing *avoidance* (profile), *undoing* and *regression* (scribbles around hair and mouth), and *identification with the aggressor* (the subject is an adult).

Becca is three years younger than Elysa, and her drawings were produced during the time she was five to eight years old (see Figs. 35A–E). In Figure 35A (at age 5 years), she was intellectually beginning to attend to more than one aspect of an object at a time, representing static realistic figures, artistically using color non-representationally and showing the first signs of a pictorial schema. The defenses manifested are *imitation, denial* and *regression. Projection* of the self and *isolation* of the objects from each other are also present. Figure 35B (at age 5.5 years) shows a quantitative difference. She was conceptualizing a slightly more complex scene containing more objects than the previous picture. Tensions appropriate during this Oedipal period are evident in the symbolic representations of mother (house) and father (sun). Elements of the pre-operational stage are seen in the portrayal of the sun with a face, an expression of magical thinking. Colors are used both non-representationally and representationally; sky and ground are illustrated, but separated, as expected for this age. Her defenses, manifested in this picture, are *projection, regression* (scribbles), *imitation* and *isolation* (unrelated forms). There is also some indication of *avoidance* and/or *undoing* in the incomplete and unrecognizable object beside the house. Figures 35C and D (at 7 years of age) show movement into the concrete operational stage. Figures are more realistic and proportions more appropriate. The defenses reflected are the same portrayed in the earlier pictures, but now include *identification* and, in Figure 35D, *identification with the aggressor*. Becca wrote on a piece of paper, which she attached to her picture, "When I grow up I will be a doctor." She drew a stethoscope on her chest. Her last picture was made when she was 8 years of age (see Fig. 35E). It is titled "self-portrait" by her mother. Becca also attached a story to this projection of herself, in which she stated that she washed dishes and wants to be an artist. Cognitively and artistically, she was more aware of realistic details, could attend to many aspects of something at the same time, and had greater control of the media. Her written words express her striving for identification with mother, but her self-portrait clarifies her anxiety surrounding this issue. There are no specific female (or for that matter male) characteristics. She chose to use the bottom of the paper to cut off the figure at an approximation of the genital area. She could draw eyes and eyelashes and other facial features skillfully, which makes one wonder about the omitted fingers in her figure. Becca appeared to be utilizing a considerable degree of *denial, isolation of affect* and *regression*. It seems that this child was moving through the post-Oedipal phase more slowly than she did in the transition from pre-operational to concrete operational functions. At the time these drawings were produced, there was no glaring evidence for concern. As stated in several sections previously, children move through sequences at their own pace and may advance in one domain more rapidly than in another. Such inconsistencies, however, should be noted and should alert parents and teachers to closely observe developmental progress.

Dayna, the third child in the family, was born one year after Becca. Drawings produced by her at four, six, seven, eight, and nine years of age will be presented (see Figs. 36A–E). At four years, Dayna was still drawing shapes within shapes, but within those shapes a figure with all its parts can be discerned (see Fig. 36A). In light of that capability, it may be inferred that her cognitive development was close to age appropriate. The encapsulation and scribbling over of forms points to the use of *regression, denial* and *undoing*.

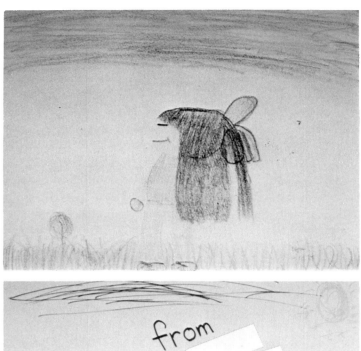

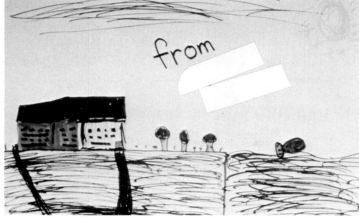

Figures 34A & B. Elysa was eight years, five months old when she drew the top picture and was nine years, five months old when she drew the bottom picture. Although a year apart, they represent overlapping developmental aspects and are age appropriate in all three domains. Defenses illustrated are isolation, identification, avoidance, along with earlier ones of projection and imitation, indicating that she has many available defenses for coping.

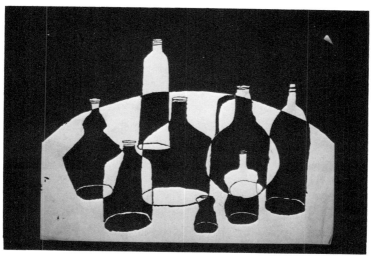

Figure 34C. Elysa, at ten years of age when she created this, reflects intellectualization and ability to execute complex images in an advanced level of cognitive and artistic development. Manifestations of doing and undoing and isolation of affect as major defenses at that time are not unusual in the pre-adolescent.

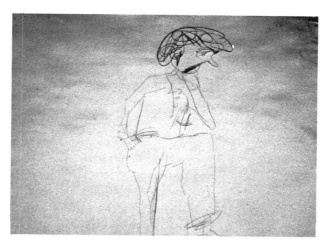

Figure 34D. Elysa, ten years old, manifests normal pre-adolescent concerns around body image in the lack of clear differentiation of sex characteristics, and at the same time her sophisticated rendering reflects her high level of intellectual and artistic performance. Defenses depicted are drawn from an earlier stage, including avoidance, undoing, and regression.

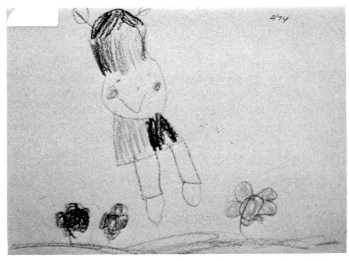

Figure 35A. Becca, five years old, draws images that attest to her ability to handle and master developmental tasks inherent in that period in all three domains. Defenses portrayed are imitation, denial, regression, projection and isolation.

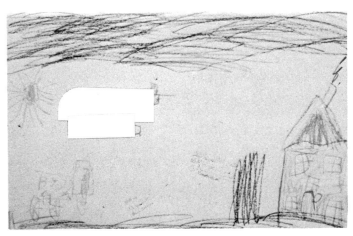

Figure 35B. Becca, five years, five months old, is now drawing a more complex scene than at five years and symbolically represents normal tension-producing objects in the environment. There is evidence of both pre-operational and concrete operational indicators of cognitive development, and defenses seen represent normal utilization at this age of projection, regression, imitation and isolation.

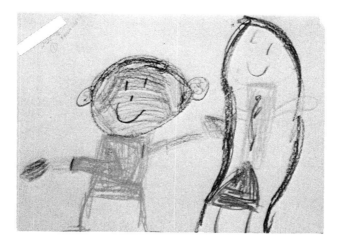

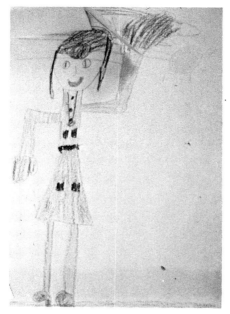

Figures 35C & D. Becca, seven years old, shows normal progression of cognitive and artistic development in these two drawings. Defenses illustrated include the ones seen in earlier figures and identification and identification with the aggressor which are both anticipated at this age.

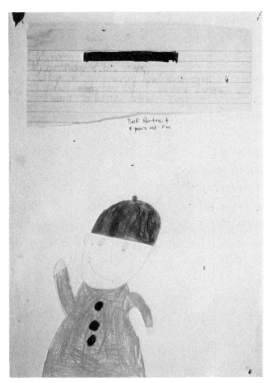

Figure 35E. Becca, eight years old, produced this self-portrait and in written words expressed a normal desire to identify with mother, which is not supported by the image. Previous skills of thinking and drawing are still present and even advanced, but the fusion of female and male characteristics in the one figure suggests anxiety around issues of identification, and the representation of immature defenses of regression, denial, and isolation are evident. Development in the three domains is not consistent with each other at this time.

At age six years, Dayna moved rapidly from pre-operational to concrete operational thought processes. Artistically, she was able to create an image that tells a story without verbal clarification (see Fig. 36B). Dayna drew a balloon carrying five people up into space, and the largest and most completely drawn figure is smiling. She described the image as "something that will make me happy," documenting her graphic fantasy. There are two large figures and three small ones. Knowing she is the third child, it is not difficult to guess that she had spontaneously drawn a family picture. Knowing also that another child was born when she was two years old, it becomes apparent that she omitted one member from the picture. The major defense manifested here is *identification with the aggressor*. Both parents can be perceived as aggressors during this period, and in the tiny rendering of the figures it is difficult to differentiate male from female. There is some scribbled filling in of the two other small balloons, implying the controlled use of *regression*. The lines in the large balloon are not scribbles. Dayna used a pen to draw her picture and had to work very hard and very carefully to fill in that space with the fine line of the medium. The utilization of *undoing* as a defense could not be determined from the picture, but knowledge of the missing sibling implies this omission was a way of *undoing* and *denying* his existence. Dayna continued her rapid progression and at seven years of age demonstrated her expanding capabilities in all areas (see Fig. 36C). The organization of her picture, spatial relationships, movement, and use of color are all more advanced than in the previous picture. Her major defense here, and appropriate for this age, was *identification*. There is no doubt that the figure is feminine. The use of *denial* is seen in the smallness of the body compared to the size of the head. It is expected that there would be denial of sexuality as well as *repression* during latency. In addition to the dress, Dayna highlighted femininity only in the facial features. Figure 36D (at age 8 years) appears to be an illustration for a story written for school. In spite of the limits on spontaneity in such a situation, Dayna solved the problem in a manner that communicates age-appropriate interest in her environment. She detailed the area around her house, and the objects in the area all loom larger than she. Interestingly enough, the story about her after-school activities does not convey the *isolation* manifested in the drawing. *Isolation of affect* is also seen in the dark holes which appear repeatedly in the trees. The tree encircled by the path is reminiscent of her earlier drawing of shapes within shapes and is a good example of the transformation of primitive forms into realistic representations. The picture shown in Figure 36E, Dayna's last picture and produced when she was nine years of age, recalls Scott's picture (see Fig. 16D) drawn when his father was out of town. There is no information as to how this picture came about. To produce such an intricate network of patterns required an advanced level of intellectual and artistic skill. In these areas, Dayna was certainly age appropriate or perhaps higher. The lower part of the picture, however, is inconsistent, and the hint of *undoing* as a defense (suggested in the discussion of Figure 36B) appears again in the totally different style of coloring in this section. The entire picture is an *avoidance* and/or *denial* of reality. It also is a projection of the "inner screen" described earlier by Noy. This pressured attempt to make order out of some feeling of disorder would not be unnatural in a pre-adolescent girl.

The next two children, whose drawings collected over time will be discussed, are brothers, sons of professional parents, and have been in close proximity to this author since their birth. From the time they were old enough to hold a pencil, both boys have been prolific artists. Brent, the older of the two, drew Figure 37A when he was six years old. All of the cognitive and artistic developmental achievements of this age are exhibited in his drawing. His creative use of material to clothe the figures is well into the concrete operational stage. *Identification* as a positive resolution of the Oedipal conflict and a defense is visible in the almost identical fashion of his own and his father's representations. He did not deny his brother Keith's existence and even shared some of father's characteristics (i.e. pants, hat and belly button). To compensate for his brother's smallness, Brent gave him an extra tall hat, which suggests the use of *reversal* and the beginning of *reaction formation*. What is particularly interesting is that although Brent has all of father's features except the belly button, he also has two of mother's. He drew the same nose for himself and his mother and colored in only the upper torso of her body and his. This contained *regression* (in the latter) and its expressive manifestation is not surprising at this age. Brent was in the process of learning that mother cannot belong to him the way she belongs to father, but the wish to be close to her was still there. Brent could have had all the material he wanted, but he chose to use it to cover only the lower parts of the figures and this covering over suggests *repression* was becoming effective. Figure 37B was produced by Brent at age seven-and-one-half years. Fantasies and preoccupation with science-fiction subjects were consonant with the interests of his peers. His underwater world is replete with "earth transporter" and "earth police station," cognitively and artistically. Defenses manifested are *denial, isolation of affect,* and *repression* and are consonant

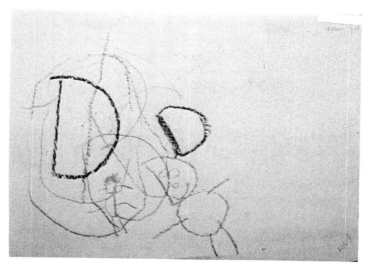

Figure 36A. Dayna, four years old, is in transition in her artistic development, drawing early shapes within shapes and figures with all the parts. Cognitive development appears appropriate and defenses are regression, denial, and undoing.

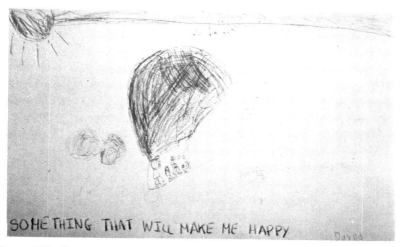

Figure 36B. Dayna, at six years of age, drew her image of "something that will make me happy." Her artistic skills give evidence of increased dexterity and cognitive conceptualization. The major defense represented is identification with the aggressor.

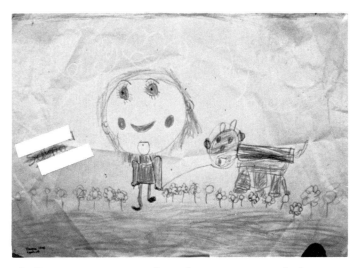

Figure 36C. Dayna, at seven years of age, demonstrates normal advancement in all three domains, and the appropriate major defense manifested here is identification. She also reflects some utilization of denial and repression, both normal at this age.

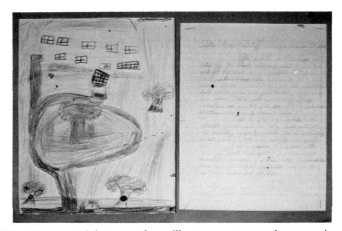

Figure 36D. Dayna, at eight years of age, illustrates a story and communicates age-appropriate interest in her environment. The rendering of the tree and path is a good example of the transformation of primitive forms (i.e. shapes within shapes) into realistic images. The drawing reveals the use of isolation and isolation of affect as a way of coping not evident in her written words.

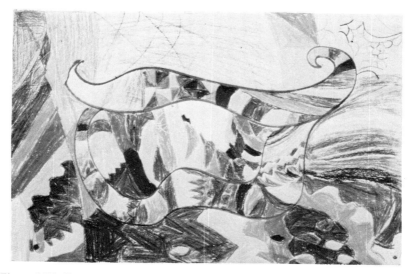

Figure 36E. Dayna, nine years old, drew this image similar to the one produced by Scott in Figure 29. It points to her advanced intellectual and artistic capabilities. Major defenses depicted are avoidance and denial, with some evidence of undoing, all of which are expected to be employed by the pre-adolescent girl at different times.

with the subject matter described previously. At age seven years, seven months, Brent illustrated his perception of Halloween (see Fig. 37C). It is difficult to see in the reproduction, but in order to include all of the images he attached several pieces of paper together and drew and cut out a number of the objects before placing them in strategic points in the picture. His ability to project his "inner screen," to symbolically and intellectually organize and transform it, visually displays his rapid progression from early to late concrete operational function. His defenses are *isolation of affect* (isolated spots of color/feeling), *reversal* (the blocked door), and *rationalization*. The first is a defense frequently observed in his behavior. The last is often expressed verbally and is evident in the depiction of the flying witch (i.e. something that a witch can do only on Halloween).

Keith, three-and-one-half years younger than Brent, was capable at four years of age of projecting his own perception of Spring, the subject of an art activity in nursery school. He could appropriately

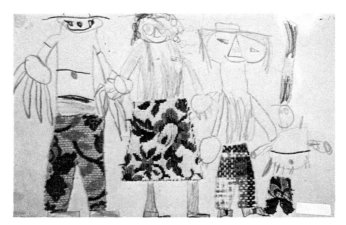

Figure 37A. Brent, six years old, is well into the concrete operational stage of cognitive development, and his two-dimensional creation of the family portrait indicates advanced artistic skills. Identification is the major defense manifested along with an example of reversal and an indication of early use of reaction formation.

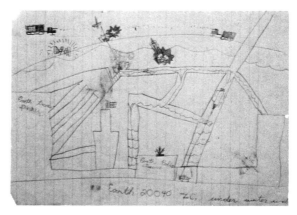

Figure 37B. Brent, at seven years, five months, illustrates fantasies and preoccupation with science fiction subjects consistent with his age group. His "underwater world" creation in a detailed line drawing confirms his progression along cognitive and artistic developmental lines. Defenses represented graphically are denial, isolation of affect and repression, all appropriate for this period of psychosexual development.

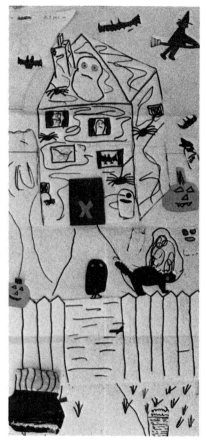

Figure 37C. Brent, at eight years, seven months, drew his perception of Halloween. This highly symbolic and intellectual visual image shows his rapid progression from early to late concrete operational function. His pictorial representation of defenses now includes rationalization.

symbolize and represent objects not present in the immediate environment. In the Oedipal phase of development, he utilized *denial of reality* in the process of expressing graphically his mental non-representational image of the assigned season (see Fig. 38A). At four years, seven months, he demonstrated his ability to attend to more than one thing at a time and pictorially depicted a schema (see Fig. 38B). He integrated opposite ideas (sun and rain) and in the process

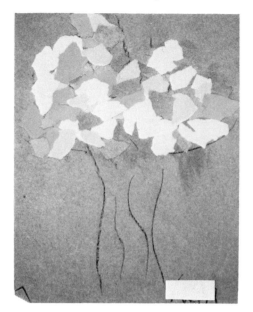
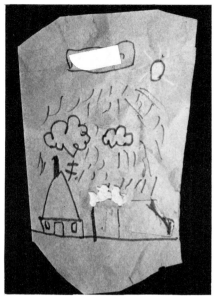

Figure 38A. Keith, four years old, projects his perception of Spring and appropriately symbolizes and represents objects not present in the immediate environment. Consistent with the pre-Oedipal phase of development, he reflects the use of denial as a defense.

Figure 38B. Keith, at four years, seven months old, is moving into the pictorial stage artistically, draws symbolic images associated with the phallic period and now manifests isolation of affect in his repertoire of defenses. Cognitively, he is able to attend to more than one aspect of something simultaneously.

used *denial of reality* to allow for their simultaneous representation. His picture displays symbols for mother and father, and, consistent with knowledge of that age, these symbols are anticipated in the drawings of the Oedipal child. He utilized *isolation of affect*, rather than *isolation*, and surprisingly this was not manifested in his behavior. On the contrary, and unlike his brother, he was known to express his feelings effectively most of the time. His last two pictures were the culmination of a Sunday school project and were produced at age five years (see Figs. 38C & D). Directed to illustrate the story of the Creation, he chose to make a booklet with a page for each day. Figure 38C is day six and shows the creation of Adam and Eve.

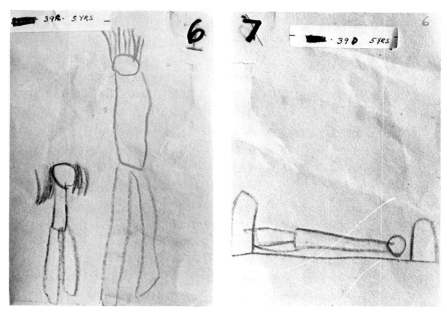

Figures 38C & D. Keith, at five years of age, made a booklet to illustrate the story of Creation, and these two drawings are days six and seven. Day 6 is the creation of Adam and Eve, and he is able to suggest some male and female characteristics. Day 7 he described as "God is resting" and is an example of concrete graphic representation. Defenses represented visually in both drawings are denial, avoidance, imitation and early identification.

There is an expression of *denial* and *avoidance* in the omission of features and some body parts. It is possible he was still concerned with projecting balance, but he nevertheless managed to suggest sex-role differentiation by the different sizes of the two figures, different head detail, and different color (still non-representational) for each figure. Keith was certainly using *imitation* and early *identification*, but still connected to both parents. On page seven, Keith drew a man lying in bed and told his teacher and mother, "God is resting," a marvelous example of a concrete graphic representation (see Fig. 38D). Depicting God as anything but a man would be total denial of his striving towards a positive identification and resolution of his Oedipal conflict. Other inferences regarding the manifestations of defense mechanisms cannot be made in relation to these two drawings, not because they cannot be differentiated from cognitive and artistic skills, but because the freedom of expression is bound by the limitations imposed by the task. Despite this, there is sufficient evidence to indicate he was functioning at an age-appropriate level in cognitive, artistic, and psychosexual development and utilizing adaptive defenses.

This chapter has attempted to present a picture of developmental sequences in cognitive, psychosexual and artistic domains. The interaction of these three systems is critical to the expression of any single one.

Based on training and experience and supported by current literature in the field of psychology and psychoanalysis, evidence points to a hierarchical structure of defense mechanisms of the ego. Their manifestations in the drawings of normal children have been presented, and the focus has been on their adaptive function in relation to age-appropriate behavior. Some examples gave rise to concerns about problems suggested in the drawings, but not evident in observable behavior. This has significant implication for identifying early signs of learning and/or emotional disorders and implementing some form of therapeutic intervention.

The following chapter will address the utilization of these defenses in a maladaptive process. Illustrations from disturbed children and adults will be used to show how identification of ego function vis-à-vis a developmental perspective of defense mechanisms reveals the level of functioning and interaction of the three systems at that time.

TABLE 2

Definitions and Criteria for Identifying Defenses Manifested in Graphic Productions

Definitions: Moore & Fine (1968) unless otherwise noted
Criteria: Author

Defense	Definition	Criteria
Incorporation	A type of introjection and an early mechanism in the process of identification. It connotes a change by imagined oral consumption of an object (person). This defense is usually employed by individuals with psychoses, impulsive disorders, oral character disorders and states of severe regression.	Symbols, forms, objects are encapsulated within other forms. Usually seen in graphic images which also indicate regression and are not generally differentiated from regression.
Projection	The source of a painful impulse or idea is perceived to exist in the external world.	Manifested in the earliest scribbles where some part of the self is represented in the lines and forms drawn on paper or some object symbolic or representative of the outside world. In more sophisticated drawings some characteristic, thought or feeling of the artist is attributed to some form or object other than self.
Displacement	A process in which repressed feelings for an object (person) are experienced in relation to another person who becomes a substitute for the original object.	Manifested in graphic productions in which the artist's known or perceived thoughts and feelings about one object are expressed graphically in relation to another object.
Symbolism	In the process of evolving symbols, the ego provides a way (language) to disguise the unacceptable.	Manifested in drawings through subjective graphic representations of specific objects and thoughts.

TABLE 2 (Continued)

Defense	Definition	Criteria
Isolation	A process in which ideas are split off from feelings which were originally associated. Used to avoid guilt, carry through a logical train of thought without contamination and distraction.	Manifested in the representation of objects drawn singly on a page; unconnected inappropriately to other forms on the page; ungrounded; separate in or from environment
Isolation of Affect	Same process as above	Concretely manifested in graphic images where color (an expression of feeling) is used or omitted inconsistently and erratically in depicting a specific form or object
Rationalization	An unconscious process that allows an individual to justify in a tolerable fashion, by plausible means, intolerable feelings, behavior and motives (Kolb, 1969).	Seen graphically in images that reflect an early attempt at a logical resolution to an unacceptable idea or feeling related to a specific situation or person in the environment.
Intellectualization	A process in which the ego binds instinctual drives through intellectual activity.	A more elaborate, sophisticated representation of a logical resolution to an unacceptable idea or feeling than the manifestation of rationalization.
Imitation	A less primitive defense than incorporation in the process of identification (A. Freud, 1965). This is a conscious process.	All representational images reflect imitation of objects and persons in the environment.

TABLE 2 (Continued)

Defense	Definition	Criteria
Reversal	A defense employed by the ego when an unacceptable aggressive or sexual wish is expressed and symbolically reversed or undone.	Feelings, situations, facts related to objects, people in environment represented graphically in a "reversed" form.
Denial	A primitive defense employed by the ego to keep from awareness some painful aspect of reality. Fantasy may also be utilized to erase from the mind that unwanted part of reality.	Absence of body parts and/or some realistic aspects of persons or objects in the environment where artist is known to be capable of appropriate representation.
Avoidance	A primitive and natural defense seen in normal development and utilized to keep an unconscious wish or narcissistic mortification from conscious awareness. Sexual and aggressive impulses are usually related to object of function being avoided (Eidelberg, 1968).	Graphically represented by side (profile) and/or back views of objects and people in the environment.
Introjection	Utilized in the process of identification in which the child carries out caretakers' (parents) demands as if they were his own even when parents are absent.	Assumed to be present in graphic images reflecting identification.
Undoing	A defense employed by the ego when an unacceptable aggressive or sexual wish is expressed and symbolically reversed or undone.	Graphically represented when the artist has changed the representation of an object, form or idea so that it is reversed, drastically changed or obliterated (undone).
Identification	An unconscious process of the ego in which an individual takes on one or more characteristics of another person and becomes like that person; usually a loved or admired person.	Images that graphically represent figures that reflect some aspects of the artist and those of some other object (person), real or fantasied, in the environment.

TABLE 2 (Continued)

Defense	Definition	Criteria
Identification with the Aggressor	The same process leading to identification, but coupled with fantasy. This allows for reversal of the role of the victim and identification with the real (or perceived) aggressor in the environment (A. Freud, 1966).	Represented in drawings of figures that reflect aspects of the artist and some aspects of an object or person in the environment who is perceived as the aggressor.
Regression	A defense employed by the individual when confronted with anxiety related to a specific aspect of maturation. A retreat to an earlier phase of psychosexual development and/or cognitive functioning is manifested in behavior.	Graphic productions will reflect regression when age appropriate representations of psychosexual, cognitive and artistic development are drawn side by side with lower age representations.
Repression	A process in which the ego keeps from conscious awareness an idea or feeling that may have been experienced consciously or curbed before it reached consciousness.	Inherent in images produced after age 6-7 where some aspects of sexual characteristics are omitted. Observed in drawings where known unacceptable thoughts and feelings are transformed or omitted.
Reaction Formation	This process follows repression of an unacceptable idea or feeling and replaces it in conscious awareness with one that is its opposite.	This is manifested in graphic images that reflect positive, acceptable ideas and feelings about a situation or object that is known to have been the source of (repressed) negative and/or painful ideas and feelings.

Chapter Five

MANIFESTATIONS OF DEFENSE MECHANISMS IN THE DRAWINGS OF DISTURBED CHILDREN AND YOUNG ADULTS

I could not talk
and so I drew
on the floor, with chalk,
When I was small.

I tried to tell you — you didn't know.
Poor soul!

I could not talk
and so I sketched
on paper, with charcoal,
When I was young.

I tried to show you — you didn't see.
Poor soul!

I could not talk
and so I painted
on canvas, with oil,
When I was grown.

I tried to reach you — you didn't
understand.
Poor soul!

I could not talk
and so I created
on clay, with my hands,
When I was old.

I tried, too late!
You can no longer feel what I say.

J.B.K.

This poem was written by a psychiatric nurse and presented as a gift to the author on the occasion of her leaving our mutual place of employment.

The image(s) of adaptive ego functions, with particular attention to the developmental sequence of mechanisms of defense, having been placed before the reader, it remains to examine how this can contribute to the existing psychological instruments used for assessing cognitive and psychosexual levels of development and their relationship to each other. It is believed that if the defense mechanisms employed by an individual can be located at a particular point in the developmental process, significant information about developmental difficulties and intrapsychic conflicts will be more readily available. This does not mean that the information alone is conclusive, but, it will be shown, this perspective adds another important dimension to the overall evaluation of human behavior. Some pertinent material from the literature will be reported and will be followed by a series of illustrations selected to address the issues raised here.

As noted earlier, Anna Freud believes that in order for defenses to become adaptive and not produce pathological results their use should be age adequate. As one example, she implies that denial and projection used to an extreme can lead to pathology in late adolescence or adulthood. It would follow then that these two defenses repeated in the drawings of older disturbed persons would be indicative of a maladaptive process. This has been documented many times in art therapy literature in connection with specific mental disorders. What is important here is the shift of focus from that mental disorder to the period that precipitated and fixed the utilization of certain defenses later recognized as maladaptive. This is not inconsistent with the clinical application of psychoanalytic theory. Further proposed here is that the graphic productions of disturbed individuals reveal not only the level of these defenses but also graphic data about the cognitive development and functions of that individual that may be difficult to obtain otherwise. It is a rich view of an individual showing many facets of his/her personality, including conscious and unconscious thoughts and feelings related to past, present and future.

It seems that learning problems in young children often herald the onset of emotional problems. Experience teaches that more often than not they are present at the same time to varying degrees but not identified because of inadequate test instruments. The degree to which one problem is expressed over the other frequently determines the kind of intervention proposed, sometimes to the neglect of the less obvious developmental issues. "Looking" at the whole person through his/her spontaneous drawings gives us a glimpse into the success or failure of that individual to master the steps up the developmental ladder. Greenspan points out that if separation and individuation are compromised, "a severe arrest at the level of pre-operational thinking may occur." This pre-operational thinking is typical of many borderline and psychotic disorders. Rosen concurs and relates that magical thinking, often expressed by such patients, has its roots in the animism, realism and participation aspects of pre-operational thought. He believes that there may be a direct relationship between psychopathological manifestations and the failure of an individual to progress "normally through age-appropriate stages and periods of cognitive development" (p. 229). He also suggests that a failure to differentiate between subject and object will result in impaired reality which will affect mature in-terpersonal relationships, and that an imbalance between assimila-tion and accommodation may produce "grossly dysfunctional behavior." The influence of parental direction is a critical factor in the successful passage from childhood to mature adulthood. Rosen cites Lidz (1973) who attributes the block that occurs in adolescence (in making this transition) to the egocentrism of some parents. Lidz considers this an underlying dynamic in persons who experience cognitive regression and schizophrenia. For example, if the parents have diffuse ego boundaries that deny realistic aspects, the adoles-cent is torn between validating his own perceptions and in-validating his/her parents' perceptions. Thus, issues around separa-tion and independence become conflicted and can lead to regression and schizophrenia (in Rosen, 1979). Clinicians are aware that, while this breakdown often occurs in late adolescence and early adulthood, it is the culmination of a family process fermenting for years. Unfortunately, these children often give clues that speak to the fragile quality of their ability to cope with stress but are not heard or seen until a crisis occurs. This is by no means intended to suggest that the community is not concerned. In fact, increased re-quests for presentations and consultations in the field of non-verbal communication emphasize serious and sincere community involve-ment in an attempt to identify these children and their families before it may be too late for educational and therapeutic interven-tion. It does suggest that the number of qualified professional personnel available is far too limited.

Rosen and Greenspan describe a study by Trunnel (1965) in which he tested normal adults and adult schizophrenic patients on Piagetian tasks. His results demonstrated that the normal subjects did better than the patient group. This is no surprise. Schizophrenia is known to impair logical reasoning even when a patient is in remission. Rosen objects to Trunnell's separating disturbed thinking from emotional conflicts and intrapsychic dynamics, an objection which is in complete accord with this discourse.

Horowitz (1970) for many years has been intrigued with the graphic productions of his psychotic patients and the relationship of these images to thought processes and defenses. He does not believe that thought processes involved in image formation are available to conscious evaluation. He reports further that the occurrence of "unbidden images" takes place despite conscious and deliberate efforts to dismiss them. His work, which investigated the underlying cognitive dynamics of unbidden images, reveals that subjectively unbidden images result from interactions between impulsive and defensive motives and reflect a "failure in repression." In terms of defenses, he concludes that repression is unsuccessful where unbidden images persist. Evidence of this has been illustrated in the drawings of post-Oedipal/latency children who are still manifesting images which should have been transformed or repressed by around age seven and after the resolution of the Oedipal conflict. These vivid (unbidden) images are like perceptions and are perceived as "unpleasant aspects of the outer world rather than as a dangerous part of the inner world," and this "extrusion of the image from the concept of self is a projective operation" (p. 168). Horowitz states that denial is also used when repression fails as a way of protecting the self from awareness of the "image formation process" and the meaning of images. This defense was seen in combination with repression in the illustrations discussed in the preceding chapter and will be more explicitly revealed in the drawings of emotionally disturbed individuals. Isolation or splitting is manifested where conflicted emotions exist. Symbolization and displacement serve to disguise ideas and feelings, and bland images often accompany expression of unpleasant feelings. Horowitz (1979) also reports that no emotion is expressed in relation to the manifestation of "horrible or lurid images." An intense example of this was a drawing produced by a patient, in treatment with me. The young woman, eighteen years of age, had been sexually abused by her stepfather when she was fourteen years old. In the course of art psychotherapy, an art psychotherapy intern encouraged her to externalize some of her debilitating rage through the safe and controlled vehicle of crayon on paper. She completed a static black line drawing of one figure stabbing another. Neither the drawing nor her verbal description of it (killing her stepfather) displayed any feeling that might be naturally, or even unnaturally, associated with this thought and image.

Examples of early manifestations of defense mechanisms in children's drawings indicating the beginning of a maladaptive process and examples of this process in advanced stages follow. In keeping with the established format, information about individuals will be disguised and related only in that it pertains to this subject and the illustration under discussion.

Illustrations

The first three examples were made available through the cooperation and interest in our work of several nursery school directors in this country and abroad.

Kim was five-and-one-half years old when he drew this picture of a house (see Fig. 39). Historical data reports that he was in an orphanage until age three at which time he was adopted, that he had considerable difficulty playing with the other children, and could rarely pay attention to a structured group activity. In addition to attending nursery school, he saw a therapist on a weekly basis, and a volunteer aide was assigned to "stay with him" throughout the nursery school hours. He was not encouraged to use art media to express or channel his frequent explosive behavior because it seemed that his mother frequently demanded he draw at home and was critical of his productions. The staff, supported by some results of psychological testing, considered him very bright but seriously disturbed. This single drawing was produced during isolated play in the kitchen. He was talking about "houses," and M, his volunteer attendant, asked him if he could draw a house. He chose the magic markers and the paper and quickly executed the image and then returned to his play. This drawing indicates that he certainly could imitate and project at least a stereotype of this object, including

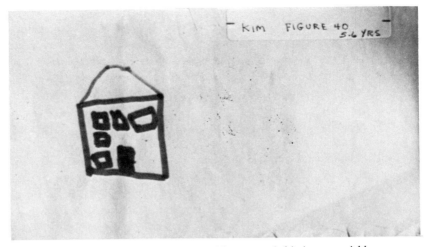

Figure 39. Kim, five years, six months old, executed this image quickly upon request. The details consistent with reality suggest he is capable of functioning
cognitively and artistically on his age-appropriate level. This image was reported
typical of his drawings and depicts the use of denial and isolation as major defenses,
which when used predominantly at this age are maladaptive.

more than one aspect of it (i.e. roof, windows, door). This is age appropriate cognitively and artistically, and to some degree, given his
attention to detail, one would expect him to be drawing pictorial
schemata. Available information about drawing done at home
reported similar productions (i.e. single, detailed objects or designs).
The defenses here mirror the manner in which he coped with objects
and people in his environment. He *denied* that environment and
isolated himself and that which may have some meaning to him at a
particular moment.

Brian was two years of age when he was referred to the nursery
where I met him. At the time of our meeting, he was four years,
three months old and had a history of echolalia, which had become
less prevalent over the past year, and he was heard to use the appropriate pronouns for himself and others more frequently. He was the
only child of an "immature" mother (case worker's description) who
was separated from his father before Brian's birth. Brian enjoyed

drawing and painting whenever there was free time. Following are two of his many drawings representative of the limited but widely diverse images he repeated over and over. Figure 40A is a "cement truck," a significant toy and symbol for some source of tension that had to be mastered. Later it was learned that the truck reflected a point of contention between the child and his mother. There was no information that made it clear if she approved or disapproved of the toy and his repeated drawings of it. It was clear, however, that he needed to be reassured I was not angry when he drew this form. He did not begin to draw until I registered my acceptance and pleasure of it at the beginning of our few meetings. This image has all the criteria to judge it age appropriate cognitively and artistically. Such aspects as the ground line and the detailed proportions all indicate that Brian was approaching concrete operational functions. The defenses in the picture are *imitation* (a mental representation of an object in the environment), *isolation* (truck is in empty environment) and *regression* (in the scribbled smoke). After completing the body of the truck, he became so influenced by the actual body movement of producing the smoke that his lines went off the edge of the page, suggesting further regression and fragile ego boundaries. The one picture would not be sufficient to warrant any inferences to suggest severe impairment. The use of isolation and regression do demand a further review of other drawings if possible, and in this case there were many available. Figure 40B is a picture of "Brian crying" and alone is cause for concern, but more so when contrasted with Figure 40A. There is no visible evidence of the level of development displayed in the image of the cement truck. The figure is grossly immature for a four year old, and the tear is totally out of proportion to the featureless face. The ability for realistic representation seen in Figure 40A directs attention not only to its absence here but also the fact that his self-image is submerged by anxiety. In discussing the picture with a member of the staff, the question of castration anxiety arose. Such anxiety is natural in the Oedipal boy, but our opinion was that this child has not reached the Oedipal period psychosexually. *Regression, denial* and *isolation*, all primitive defenses, are manifested. Decarie (1962), cited by Greenspan, maintains regression will occur when the symbiotic pressures are too great, and the representational capacity will be blunted. Brian had not reached the level of development to sense a fear of castration; he was overwhelmingly fearful of annihilation. His depiction of himself (repeated in other drawings produced in the nursery), the defenses evoked, all imply that emotionally he had not dealt successfully with separation and individuation and psychosexually was still attached symbiotically to his mother. He was not yet whole, and he tearfully communicated his fear that he will never be complete. These "educated guesses" were borne out by his therapist (who met with him for a short period of time every day), who further validated in his report that Brian's mother had as much difficulty separating from him as he did from her. The contrast in his levels of development in the two domains (cognitive + psychosexual) is an excellent example of Greenspan's view of the internal and external boundaries out of harmony. This disharmony, at this age, leads one to hold a dim view for Brian's future capacity to attain any satisfactory level of equilibrium. Of interest also is the knowledge that his capabilities cognitively contradict the results of a study reported by Greenspan. The investigators, Blatt, Allison and Baker (1965), concluded that persons who had not resolved conflicts "over body integrity or with poor body image" cannot perform well on "cognitive tasks demanding ability to assemble wholes from parts presented visually." Their task was the Wechsler Object Assembly Subtest (p. 133). Contrary to their findings, Brian was capable of putting puzzles together with the same dexterity as the other four and five year olds. This points out the danger in making generalizations from limited studies even though there is strong evidence in the literature and full agreement here with the developmental relationship between cognitive and psychosexual growth. This very relationship and interaction, when understood, explain some reasons for the differences in development.

Michael at four years, ten months of age could also do puzzles, but only when his nursery school teacher sat with him and guided the activity by pointing out colors in pieces that were the same as sections of the picture showing the completed puzzle. Michael seemed aware that he should be able to do better by himself and became frustrated in this situation and others, which led to explosive behavior. He rightfully worried his teacher. The perceptive, sensitive, and caring woman was concerned that Michael would have serious emotional problems in public school, which by law he was required to enter within two months. During my visit to the nursery, Michael joined a group of children drawing with me and also began

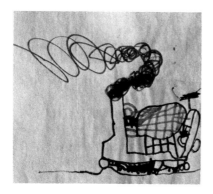 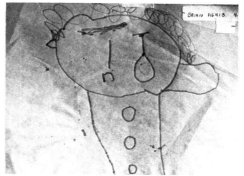

Figures 40A & B. Brian, at four years, three months old, produced these two drawings within a few days. He called the picture on the left a "cement truck" and the one on the right was a picture of "Brian crying," and together they reveal differences between cognitive and psychosexual development. On an intellectual level, he is approaching the concrete operational level, whereas his image of self is typical of images drawn by a two- to three-year-old child. This developmental disharmony causes him to have only primitive defenses at his disposal and those illustrated are regression, denial, and isolation.

to draw. This drawing is not available for reproduction. I was not engaged in evaluating any of the children's drawings for any purpose but was immediately struck by the bizarre quality of his imagery. He said it was a house with a staircase, and his representation of it was far below a four- to five-year-old level. The shaky lines and the slanting of the entire image led me to challenge the assumption that all of his problems were functional, but from the history there was good reason to believe this assumption. He is an adopted child (and had recently learned this), the younger of two boys. The older son is the natural child of a couple who for the past two years had experienced extreme marital discord, including several separations and reconciliations. At the time under discussion, Michael's father had been away from home for almost a year, rarely seeing his sons. In spite of this traumatic environment, I believed Michael had a perceptual problem that was organic, and further testing was recommended. He had been tested several months previously, but the examination did not include psychological testing instruments, such as the Bender Gestalt, because they are not part of the routine evaluating procedure at that school. Subsequently, in the interest of time, I was approached to do an art therapy evaluation of Michael to see if there was, in fact, consistent evidence of minimal brain dysfunction. Figures 41A, B, and C are the drawings produced during that evaluation, and they confirmed my original suspicions, which were later validated by the school psychologist. The subject of diagnostic indicators in drawings of organic brain syndromes is an aspect of art therapy that was not originally intended for this study. It is presented here, briefly, because the line between manifestations of organic and functional disorders is sometimes so fine that the untrained eye could easily misread the clues, especially where historical data seem to strongly point to one source of the disorder. The three evaluation tasks assigned were a free drawing, a house and a person. This is not a typical art therapy assessment but was tailored to allow Michael as much freedom from pressure as possible and at the same time to provide a broad enough range of images upon which to base further recommendations. Throughout the test, Michael was aware that these were "not like" what they were supposed to be, and he needed a great deal of encouragement to complete each drawing. The first picture was a car, begun with the two wheels (see Fig. 41A); the second picture was a house, as directed (see Fig. 41B), and the third picture was of a man who "was cross" (see Fig. 41C). There was no doubt that Michael was showing clinical signs of emotional disturbance (believed by the staff to be the sole cause of present and anticipated problems). This conclusion was partially correct, but was now compounded by the fact that Michael also had an organic learning disorder. The expressions of defense mechanisms in his drawings are primitive and limited. Michael used *denial* (omission of body parts and fantastical distortions), *isolation* (images suspended in space and/or unconnected to other images in the picture), *regression* and *undoing* (the isolated scribbling and scribbling over lines and objects) throughout his productions.

There is also *reversal* in the image of the man who, described as cross, is smiling. The picture shown in Figure 41D was done several days later while we were sitting together. He started with the bottom part, then added the first figure on the left who was himself "shooting and killing robots with his ray gun." I asked him if he could draw his family, and apparently he was comfortable with my expectations and added a second figure. He said this was Tom (his brother), who was not shooting because "the robot was his best friend." The third figure was his father who was "not seeing" and therefore "not shoot-ing." He told me he would not add his mother because "she would get hurt." In spite of his perceptual handicap, the same defenses pre-vailed and were supported by his associations and comments. He *de-nied* his father's absence from home and omitted the mother, osten-sibly to protect her. He was denying his anger at her (it is his pic-ture, and who else would shoot her?) and at the same time *reversing* that feeling to one of concern and caring. Predicting any prognosis is always a difficult psychological venture. Nevertheless, it was be-lieved that this child would do well with a specialized school pro-gram and therapy for him and his mother. In denying his father's absence, he was also struggling to *identify* with him as well as with his older brother. The figure drawings do indeed reflect Michael's poor self-image, but the complete representation of that and any other image was in part hampered by his perceptual difficulties. His mother, it was learned, was managing to cope with her problems and to address Michael's. Arrangements were made for him to receive special tutoring and to see a therapist once a week. Michael is an interesting contrast to Brian (see Figs. 40A and B), and there is greater concern for Brian's future in spite of his advanced intellec-tual capacity.

Figures 42A, B and C were brought to me for an evaluation by a therapist who, on occasion, utilizes drawings in her clinical practice. The drawings were subsequently offered (and gratefully acknowl-edged) for this work. GB was eight years old when she was referred for treatment because of emotional problems. Figure 42A was done spontaneously during a therapy session and reflects an age-appropriate representation of a human figure, both cognitively and artistically. *Isolation* and *denial* and *regression* are exhibited, but the non-representational use of color and the regression, suggesting *un-doing*, reflect her anxiety about her self-image. One hand is raised as if to ward off some danger, and the entire figure, particularly the gaping, toothy mouth, imparts *identification with the aggressor*. Figure 42B is an incredible, spontaneous drawing done by the mother at a separate time while she was waiting for her daughter to end her meeting with the therapist. The mother's drawing is more immature than the child's, but the open mouth with clenched teeth is so similar it leaves little doubt as to who the aggressor is. It suggested that this mother also identified with someone she perceived as an aggressor.

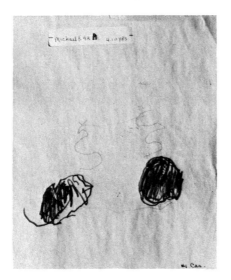

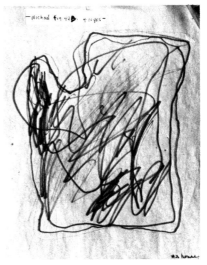

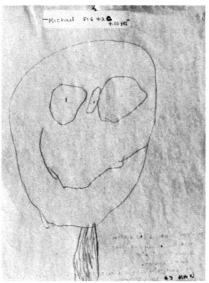

Figures 41A, B, & C. Michael, four years, ten months old, produced these drawings during an art therapy evaluation, consisting of three tasks: a free drawing, a house and a person. In addition to revealing indicators of organic brain dysfunction, Michael manifested primitive defenses of denial, regression, undoing, reversal, and isolation.

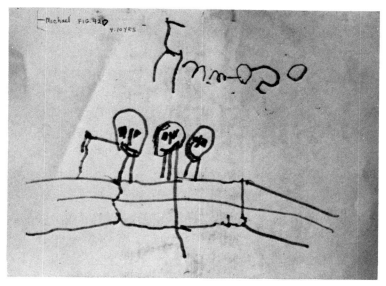

Figure 41D. Michael drew this family portrait several days after he drew the pictures in Figures 41A, B, and C and illustrates his difficulty with the developmental task of identification in the reflection of his extremely poor self-image. This, compounded by perceptual difficulties, leaves him with limited resources to cope with normal developmental stress.

Working with abused children and their parents has taught us that there is a common factor (i.e. parents of abused children have themselves been victims of abuse, and their own identification has often proceeded in that direction as a way of mastering and coping with the psychological or physical assault). As parents, they displace their rage onto their children. A year later, at age nine, and making considerable progress in therapy, GB produced Figure 42C. This is a marvelous example of splitting the good and bad perceived in one individual (in this case, mother). In Figure 42A, GB incorporated the aggressive open mouth with clenched teeth exposed from her mother's drawing (see Fig. 42B). In Figure 42C, GB incorporated the playful activity (jumping rope, seen in mother's drawing) in her projection of self. What is remarkable is that, according to the therapist, neither had any access to the other's drawings, yet this young girl replicated her mother's pictorial representation of eyes (a definitely feminine characteristic) and now used her arms to jump

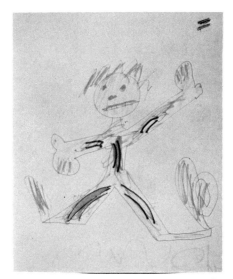 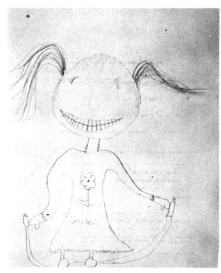

Figure 42A. The picture shown on the left was done by GB, eight years old, who did this drawing spontaneously during a therapy session. Artistically and cognitively, she is functioning on an age-appropriate level, but illustrated defenses of isolation, denial, regression, undoing, and identification with the aggressor reflect concerns about body image and are not typical for this age (courtesy of GB's therapist, Ms. A.).

Figure 42B. The picture shown on the right was done by GB's mother (age not known), who drew this spontaneously while waiting for her daughter. Her image indicates that she is functioning on a cognitive, artistic and psychosexual level around the age of five years (courtesy of GB's therapist, Ms. A.).

rope like her mother. Cognitively and artistically, she incorporated a ground line and used color more representationally. *Identification* was utilized in a more adaptive manner, and there is no evidence of *regression* or *undoing*. The reversal of the angry mouth to the smiling one may also mirror the beginning of *reaction formation*. The *isolation* here is made less obvious by the grounding of the figure, which creates a much more solid image than the previous floating one.

In the foregoing illustrations, we have examined the manifestations of fixed, rigid defenses in children's drawings, inhibiting growth towards a mature, flexible synthesis of internal and external influences and boundaries. Let us now consider how these defenses

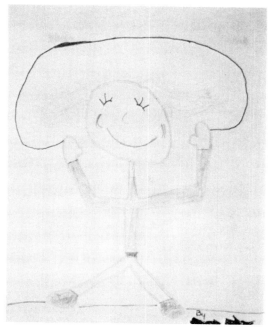

Figure 42C. GB, nine years of age, spontaneously produced this image, and the similarity to Figure 43A is noted. Cognitively and artistically, she used color more representationally and included a ground line. Defenses manifested now include identification, and there is no evidence of regression or undoing (courtesy of GB's therapist, Ms. A.).

are manifested first in the graphic productions of neurotic patients, then in those of psychotic patients. Only a few examples will be given. We continue to frown upon generalizations, but, if one accepts psychoanalytic theory regarding the conflicted and unresolved stages of psychosexual development in which these mental disorders originate, it follows that the defense mechanisms employed by the individuals in the examples would be consistent with that period of development. Their manifestations in drawings often lead to recognition of the point of fixation before it is identifiable clinically and they present a coherent picture of the mental status of the individual at that time. Spontaneous drawings also reveal cognitive development which must be considered along with affectual development in order to determine treatment goals. For example, Greenspan reports that neurotic structures have elements of concrete and pre-operational thinking. For some neurotic patients, separation and individuation may still be incomplete and identification tenuous.

Robert was twenty years old and a second-year art student when he was referred for treatment of overwhelming anxiety and suicidal ideation. Figures 43A and B are two of a series of six produced in the early months of treatment. They are significant because symbolically they represented his feelings of being trapped and unable to free himself of parental ties and dominance. He had chosen a school two thousand miles away from home but soon realized that physical distance did little to sever the strong psychological connection. His initial drawings produced in the first month of therapy were highly structured, tightly drawn, realistic pictures and displayed his intellectual capacity to organize and conceptualize objects and people in his environment coherently, but with little affect. Those early drawings quickly pointed to an obsessional neurosis, carrying with it the need to isolate feelings from thoughts. This conclusion is based on the author's years of experience working with obsessional patients in art therapy. Intense and repeated encouragement was necessary before Robert would permit himself to do quick, spontaneous images. Even with this freer form of expression, the same defenses are observable. *Isolation of affect, undoing* and controlled *regression*, all rigidly enforced for the purpose of prohibiting unacceptable thoughts and feelings related to the pre-phallic stage of development.

A distortion in character formation and what is described as a "hysterical character" (Moore & Fine, 1968) may also be the result of unresolved issues before and during the Oedipal period.

C referred himself for therapy because he was experiencing severe anxiety about an imminent change in his life (going back to college in his mid-twenties), and he was aware that he frequently "acted out." All of this was related in a highly intellectualized and emotionless manner. Art psychotherapy soon revealed a major conflict centered around the process of identification, while another deeper one revolved around separation and individuation. C was in therapy for several years, his dynamics were complex and his graphic productions are discussed in depth in a paper on transference and countertransference (1975). His *intellectualization* remained for a long

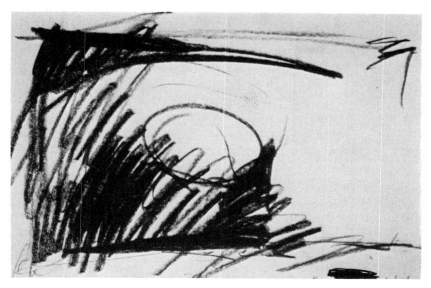

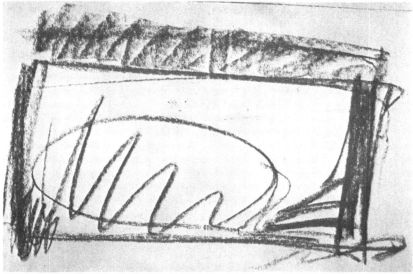

Figures 43A & B. Robert, twenty years old, did these two drawings during art psychotherapy sessions. They are typical of many he did over a six-month period. Consistent and repeated manifestations of defenses of isolation of affect, undoing, and controlled regression identified his intrapsychic conflict as emanating from the pre-phallic stage of development.

time his primary defense in verbal communication and was well supported by a highly advanced repertoire of cognitive skills. The latter served him well in the organization and control of his graphic images, but his defense mechanisms of *isolation, denial, reversal* and *avoidance* remained fixed (see Figs. 44A & B). Figure 44A is an early symbolic representation of his mother, a box-like form with compartmentalized body parts. Figure 44B is a picture of the "therapist watching the patient in a fish bowl." Looking closely, one can see that the therapist's eyes are closed and that she is turned away from the fish bowl. His own wish to be equal to the therapist (expressed verbally), to be seen as he wished, is *denied* in the image, and his *avoidance* of dealing with these thoughts and feelings is *projected* onto the turned-away figure of the therapist. *Isolation* in the fish bowl is complete. C exemplifies the person described by Greenspan who has a well-developed representational capacity, which should go hand in hand with "assertiveness, mobility and stability, but remains dependent." The mature attributes have not been derived from the transformed representational capacity (p. 350).

Awareness of reality is a principal factor in differentiating neurosis from psychosis. The neurotic patient is in touch with reality, whereas the psychotic patient is not. For the psychotic patient, fantasies are often believed to be fact. The next two illustrations were done by eighteen-year-old Wilma, an acute paranoid schizophrenic patient.

Figure 45A is typical of fragmented images produced repeatedly by schizophrenic patients. The order of the forms is not haphazard and reflects in a bizarre, unrealistic way Wilma's advanced level of cognitive skills to make order out of her perceived chaotic world. *Regression* is a major defense for psychotic patients who reject reality because it is so painful and they have so few defenses with which to cope. Forms like this are a return to the pleasurable artistic period of making shapes within shapes. It is helpful to compare this image to the ones produced by Scott (see Fig. 15D) and Dayna (see Fig. 36E). Their spatial organization and relationship between forms are missing from Wilma's who, like them, was *denying* reality and *isolating* feelings, but in a much more regressive fashion. Her second picture is an image that she created whenever there was a stressful situation (see Fig. 45B). Many months after she was admitted to the hospital, the "inner screen" this image projected was uncovered by her during

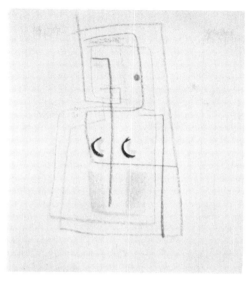

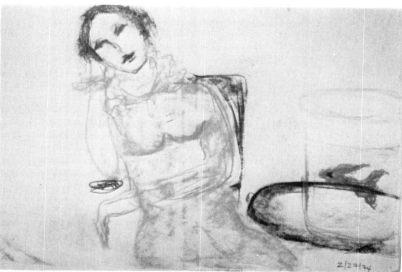

Figures 44A & B. C, twenty-three years old when he produced the top picture and twenty-five years old when he produced the bottom picture, drew both pictures during art psychotherapy sessions. The first is a symbolic representation of mother, and the second is a picture of the "therapist watching the patient in a fish bowl." In spite of his primary defense of intellectualization in verbal communication and an advanced repertoire of cognitive and artistic skills, his defenses manifested repeatedly in his imagery were isolation, denial, reversal and avoidance and indicated his psychosexual development was on a pre-phallic level.

a session with her art therapist. This was a symbolic representation of a sexual abuse at the age of seven, still *denied, isolated* and *displaced* from the lower torso to the middle torso. The long-suppressed trauma was exacerbated by an unwanted therapeutic abortion at age seventeen. The psychic energy invested in the task of keeping the earlier disruption in development repressed stripped her of whatever adaptive mechanisms she may have acquired and demanded the rigid maladaptive defenses seen in her drawings, but only suspected and surmised in her clinical withdrawal.

Figures 46A, B and C provide a cross-section of a twenty-eight-year-old woman's artistic creations during a four-year period. Diagnosed as those of a chronic paranoid schizophrenic, these images communicate the degree to which Chris was in touch with reality at the time they were done. Whether symbolic or realistic, her forms are static, *isolated* and imbued with *denial*. The flowers depict one of her rare compositions that do not contain a blatant expression of regression (see Fig. 46B). It was executed shortly after her discharge from an inpatient unit and at the beginning of a short-lived remission. The most regressed representation expressed is in Figure 46C and is symbolic of her symbiotic relationship with her mother (transferred to the therapist) and inability to separate and individuate. Prior to the onset of the illness, her IQ was assessed at 165, and when in fairly close contact with reality she could call on her intellectual skills to draw realistic representations. But invariably the images of females faced away from view and their sexual characteristics were *denied* and *avoided* (see Fig. 46A).

Finally, we have examples of two patients, who exemplify a multitude of others who spoke but were not heard until it was too late. Their stories must serve as a lesson to remind us that what we hear is not necessarily what it is.

Pat was admitted to a city mental hospital at the age of seventeen before involuntary admissions were challenged and changed by law. Her diagnosis at that young age was chronic undifferentiated schizophrenia, and the history reviewed a number of hospitalizations, inability to function in school since latency period, and explosive behavior in school and at home. Family and peers called her "crazy." She was placed in a therapeutic milieu where she was expected to participate in all group therapy and activity sessions. The explosive behavior escalated, and medication was deemed the only solution. While serving as a consultant to the unit, this author and

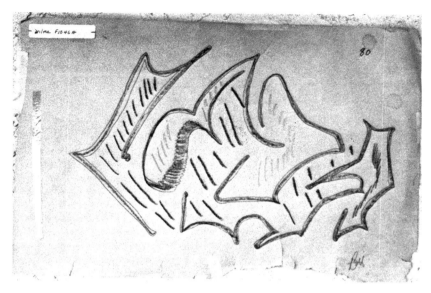

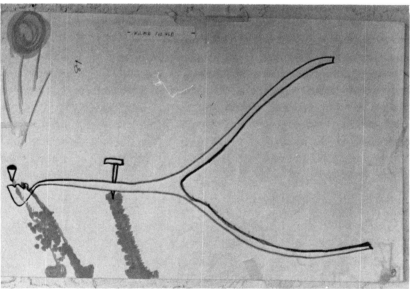

Figures 45A & B. Wilma, nineteen years old, produced these images during hospitalization for an acute psychotic episode. Regression — a primary defense utilized by psychotic patients — is seen here in the return to drawing shapes within shapes and reflects impaired cognitive and artistic functions. In the bottom picture, there is evidence of the utilization of primitive defenses of denial, isolation and displacement.

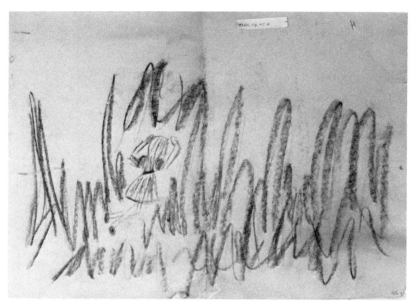

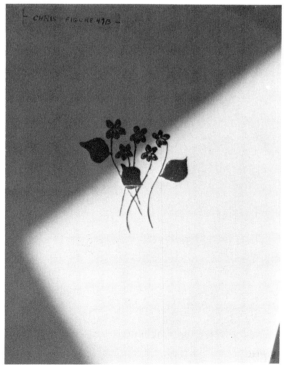

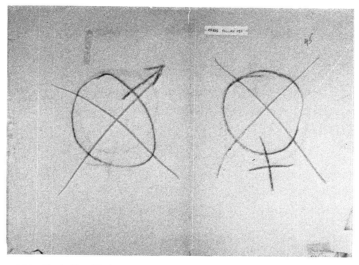

Figures 46A, B, & C. Chris, twenty-four to twenty-eight years old when she drew these pictures, was diagnosed as a paranoid schizophrenic patient. When in remission, she was capable of demonstrating advanced levels of cognitive and artistic development (such as shown in the below opposite picture), but even here her forms remain static and isolated. Her coping resources were limited, and her drawings repeatedly revealed the early defenses of regression, denial, isolation, and avoidance.

staff art therapist reviewed Pat's drawings. Figures 47A, B and C are drawings that appeared at first glance to be produced by a child of about three or four years of age. The tracing of her own hand is similar to what Indira and her little friends did when we first met (see Fig. 47A). The other two drawings, when looked at more closely, showed distortions that were atypical of children's depictions. There are repeated lines and shapes that strongly suggested perseveration, associated with organic brain syndrome (see Fig. 47C), and a quality of imagery that on the one hand was very immature and on the other showed some awareness of self and objects in the environment on a more advanced level. A recommendation for a battery of psychological tests was made. The results of the multi-evaluation procedures confirmed this young woman to be brain damaged. In retrospect, it can only be guessed that perhaps she realized she could not perform in school, so frustration and shame may have provoked behaviors that eventually were labeled "crazy." At the time she was evaluated there was sufficient clinical evidence to point to a severe emotional

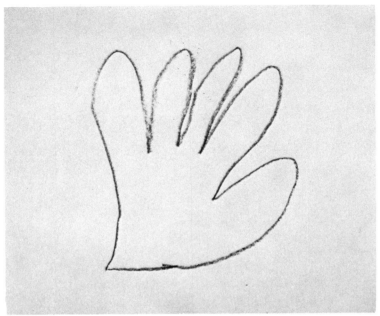

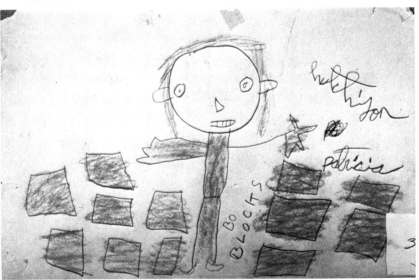

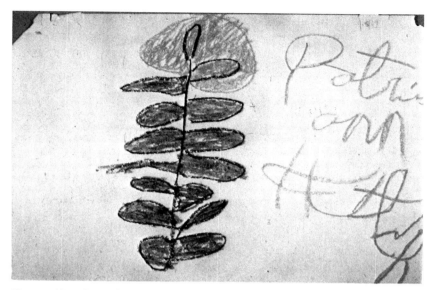

Figures 47A, B, & C. Pat, seventeen years old, was committed to a psychiatric ward with a diagnosis of chronic schizophrenia and produced these drawings in art therapy sessions during the first three weeks of her hospitalization. Her imagery supported the clinical evidence of a severe mental disorder, but also demonstrated that she was functioning on a cognitive and artistic level of about a three to four year old and also suggested brain damage. These conclusions from her graphic representations were subsequently confirmed in the results of a battery of psychological evaluations.

disorder as well, but placement in a therapeutic milieu was inappropriate for her level of mental functioning. When directed in individual "play" activities, she responded like a little child, like the girl pictured in Figure 47B.

Long ago the notion that schizophrenic patients are incapable of gaining insights was discarded and replaced with the knowledge that insights could be incorporated successfully into the therapeutic process with this population. Naumburg (1947) postulated this as a general theory of art therapy, which is in part rejected here. Along with the notion stated above, the recognition of the role cognitive skills play in this therapeutic process must be acknowledged. Chris, because of her innate intelligence, could over the years "learn" new ways to cope that were more adaptive than some of her earlier ways, taking advantage of the myriad of therapeutic endeavors. Pat had limited intellectual capacities, and to subject her to the pressure of intense psychiatric involvement was a cruel injustice and a tragic misjudgment by the community at large.

Dee's drawings tell of yet another case where the images spoke to the problems ahead, but no one heard till much later (see Figs. 48A, B, & C). Her images were lent to this author by her current art therapist. Miss L, as we shall call her therapist, was working with Dee as part of the therapeutic team on the unit where Dee, now in her twenties, had been admitted in an acute psychotic episode. Her history revealed this was a repeated experience over the years. Members of her family brought in a scrapbook containing reproductions of her drawings beginning when she was three years of age. Miss L was intrigued with the extraordinary precociousness visible at that age, and the startling changes within months, and shared them with this author. "The budding artist" at three years, nine months old could illustrate realistic figures, visually depict actions like skating, and draw excellent representations of moving vehicles (see Fig. 48A). Defenses manifested are *isolation, imitation*, early *identification*, and *displacement* of wishes and fantasies onto objects in the environment (in this case, the drawing paper). Only months later, instead of progression into organized, pictorial schemata, her images presage *regression* and decompensation of earlier structures. The colors are vivid, but non-representational; the figures are distorted in a manner unlike those drawn by children still concerned with balance (see Figs. 48B & C). Perusing some of the drawings accumulated and saved over the years, we learned that Dee poignantly speaks of her pain and subsequent withdrawal, but no one saw until the bright, creative child was out of sight. This sudden graphic expression of regression fixes the point in development when she experienced trauma, not seriously considered until her behavior much later demanded psychiatric attention.

An effort will be made in the following section to extrapolate and synthesize consequential issues from this presentation.

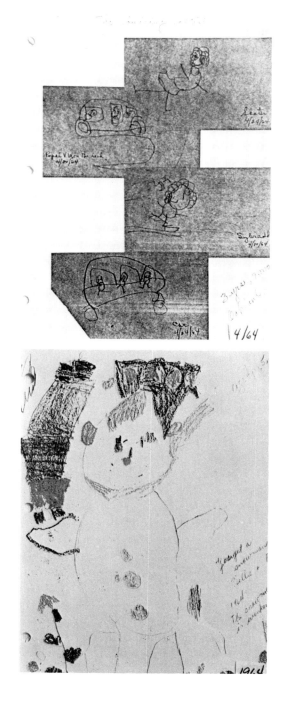

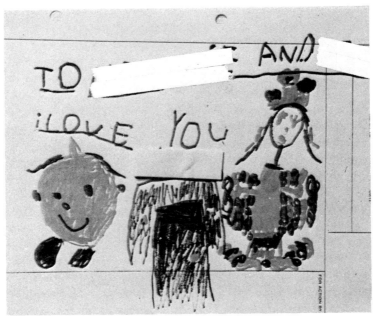

Figures 48A, B, & C. Dee, three years, nine months to four years, produced these images spontaneously in her home environment where they were preserved in a scrapbook. At age twenty, she was hospitalized for an acute psychotic episode and they were released to her therapist, Miss. L. The first drawing shows she could produce images depicting action and representing moving vehicles, indicating her cognitive and artistic development was on a much higher level than her chronological age. Defenses manifested are isolation, imitation, early identification, and displacement, and the three domains are developmentally parallel. Within a few months, her images indicate regression and decompensation of earlier higher-level representations, fixing the point in development when she experienced severe psychological trauma (courtesy of Dee's therapist, Miss. L.).

Chapter Six

CONCLUSION

REVIEWING the literature can be like sifting through a treasure chest and, unlike Pandora's box, releasing not demons but hope of positive possibilities. One treasure was discovered in the work of Arnheim, who gives a moving account of the motivation behind the magnificently expressive paintings of the well-known artist, Paul Klee. Arnheim recounts that Klee wrote in his diary, "pour ne pas pleurer: that is the first and last reason." He interprets this as evidence that the artist's creativity served as an "alternative to weeping." He also points out that this process served Klee well because it clarified for him "what there was to weep about and how one could live with, and in spite of, this state of affairs" (Arnheim, 1969, p. 254). One needs only to look at Klee's paintings to recognize his talent and intelligence. His images are symbolic condensations of the ego function of synthesis expressed through creative art. It is true that not everyone has the talent and intelligence reflected in Klee's work, so what message does he (and Arnheim) provide us? Arnheim says art is "to give visible form to all aspects of life" (p. 295). In art therapy, art is communication. The earliest graphic scribbles are projections of kinesthetic pleasure experienced by all children universally. As children develop, their images chronicle their growth, and the manifestations of this incredible human experience are the thrust of this author's work on the adaptive process. For Klee, the making of art was an adaptive process; for most not endowed with his abilities, art remains an open book that needs to be read carefully and, where necessary, clarified and interpreted for the struggling, growing child, and the suffering adult, by qualified "readers." For those who have struggled through the maze of images and discussion in the preceding chapters, many questions have surely arisen and even some frustration that obvious data emanating from the drawings about some individuals seem to have been ignored. It must be remembered that in-depth case studies were beyond the scope of the topic central to this work, and the reader is referred to the comprehensive bibliography on art therapy for numerous examples of art as a therapeutic modality. Nevertheless, some issues remain to be clarified. These were noted by the author in the process of preparing this text and will be presented in order.

One instance originates in the anal to phallic stage (2 to 3 years of age) and suggests a marked difference between a defense observed in clinical observation during a particular stage of development and one noted in a child's drawing and the drawings of an adult neurotic patient in treatment with this author.

Anna Freud reported observing *avoidance* in some children's behavior, of displeasing qualities, attitudes, smells, etc., as a natural defense in the anal stage. Indira's image of "Mr. Uppity" and patient C's image of himself in the fish bowl, both expressions of *isolation* in relation to displeasing events in their environments, suggest the use of a different defense than the one suggested by Anna Freud (i.e. avoidance). This difference requires further investigation, particularly if that defense becomes employed to any extreme degree. In Indira's case *isolation* was seen also in behavior in more stressful situations, and at times forced her withdrawal from the group (see Fig. 10). C for the most part employed both *isolation* and *avoidance* interchangeably, but did, in fact, more frequently isolate himself in a way that was tantamount to withdrawal in extreme states of depression (see Figs. 44A & B). An interesting question provoked by this difference is the relationship of the two defenses. It may be that *isolation* is a more primitive defense and therefore more observable in manifest imagery, whereas *avoidance*, a more sophisticated defense, is recognized by the child and later the adult as more socially adaptable.

Harry (see Fig. 12) and Leon (see Fig. 13) both presented inconsistencies between verbal skills and artistic development. The whole issue of language development has spurred considerable research. Some of the literature does support the idea that language and imagery develop parallel to each other. Opposing views will be formed for some time around this argument, and Harry and Leon present two separate facets of the subject. Harry, described as "an overindulged child" by one member of the staff, mirrored anger and frustration in his smeary pictures, and an outlet for his feelings is sorely needed if these defenses are not to become rigid. His capacity for articulation does not provide an adequate channel for his anger. Leon presents drawings that imply he is simply going through the artistic sequential stages very slowly, while his verbal skills progress appropriately. Explanations for these individual differences vary, and perhaps the most important thing is to recognize these differences and to be prepared to help those children with inconsistencies in their development catch up in the lagging domain by identifying and alleviating the block interfering with normal growth. Also important is how this knowledge can be used to establish realistic expectations for these children to prevent the use of inhibition as a defense that often leads to emotional problems.

The children in the classroom taught by the unusual teacher described on page 81, did not conform to two generalizations. First, figures are normally static in children's drawings in the pre-operational and early concrete stages, whereas most of the figures drawn by her two classes contained movement. This advanced level of visual representation is attributed to the fact that the children were always invited to express themselves in body movement in the process of "feeling" and "acting out" sounds. They were in touch with movement in a way that is not common in most school systems. Such an experience would be beneficial to all children.

The second area in which they differed was their wider use of the stick figure (while still expressing the movement noted above). It has been mentioned previously that there was some agreement here with Greenspan, who questioned if latency in fact was a quiescent period as traditionally considered in psychoanalytic theory. One of the reasons that this has not appeared to be so in the last ten to twelve years is thought to be the increased exposure to sexual material on television and a change in society's values. This exposure does not allow for repression of sexual fantasies to become effective. Psychoanalytic theory describes the latency period as one in which there is a moratorium on these fantasies, enabling the child to attend to the task of learning and the development of peer relationships. The community in which this author's friend teaches is a tightly knit environment with rather homogeneous ethnic and cultural traditions and rituals. It is suspected that, although television is available, some shows and movies are not considered acceptable for family viewing as readily as they might be in other urban areas of the country. Thus, repression of sexual ideation is reinforced. Another note about stick figures observed in clinical practice is that they are commonly used by adults who are asked to draw. Most people who have not drawn since their early school years find this the least-threatening way to represent a figure and rationalize its use on the basis of their lack of artistic skills. Clinically, this must be evaluated in the context in which it is produced to determine if it is indeed a denial of sexuality or symbolic avoidance of some other tension-provoking situation.

The question of style was addressed in connection with the discussion of regression and identification with the aggressor seen in the drawings of two boys (see Figs. 26 & 28). Individuals draw in different ways, which reflect their personality traits. Just as someone may be a casual or relaxed housekeeper, someone may draw in a loose, sketchy way. This is not to be confused with regression, which, as a defense, is different from one's habitual work habits.

In the concluding section of his work, Greenspan postulates the need for a comprehensive evaluation instrument that will include measures to test verbal and manual skills. This thesis attempted to demonstrate that no evaluation procedure can be comprehensive without the inclusion of spontaneous drawings. The data available from these images pertaining to numerous aspects of human behavior have been accepted and utilized by many in the field of mental health for some time.

There are many political arguments both for and against the "labeling" of individuals suffering from mental disorders, a critical forensic topic that will not be addressed here. It is incumbent, however, upon the cadre of professionally trained people committed to the field of mental health, regardless of discipline, to acknowledge that treatment must be based on some decision which constitutes a form of diagnosis. Members of different disciplines have to surrender rigid views and even traditional ways of "looking at" and defining emotional problems. No single approach to psychodiagnosis has ever proved adequate. The theory described here is meant to provide another explicit method for identifying events in the course of human development. It strongly supports the current findings that neither psychosexual nor cognitive development can be viewed separately but must be considered as two parts of a whole that are always interacting and reflecting internal and external influences in the maturational process. How one responds to these influences forms the nucleus of the ability to adapt and subsequently to allow ego functions to integrate and synthesize available resources productively within the social milieu.

Documentation has been offered showing how these adaptive aspects of the personality are clearly manifested in the graphic productions of children and adults. Maladaptive measures employed by individuals in the face of trauma or genetic impairment have also been demonstrated. Locating these adaptive and/or maladaptive defenses at a particular point in development has enormous implication in the early intervention and treatment of mental disorders. It may also alleviate in some small measure a number of those children who are mistakenly diagnosed in the early school years (i.e. considered behavior problems when in fact they are brain damaged).

Members of education and mental health disciplines, other than art therapists, can use graphic productions to discern whether or not a child or an adult has age-appropriate capabilities. In the absence of some or all of those criteria, a mental flag should be raised to call for further evaluation by qualified art and other psychodiagnosticians.

Arnheim, a brilliant investigator in the fields of education and art, beautifully summarizes the relationship between thinking and perception in the "implicit assumption that every artwork is a statement about something." And the function of art can now be recognized in general education if "it is recognized that productive thinking in any area of cognition is perceptual thinking" (p. 296). This, coupled with the imagery of parallel perceptions related to psychosexual development, provides the knowledgeable evaluator of spontaneous and even directed drawings with a sensitive serviceable schema.

He always wanted to explain things,
   but no one cared.
So he drew.
Sometimes he would draw and it wasn't anything .
He wanted to carve it in stone or write it in the sky.
He would lie out on the grass and look up in the sky.
And it would be only him and the sky and the things
   inside him that needed saying.
And it was after that he drew the picture.
It was a beautiful picture.
He kept it under his pillow and let no one see it.
And he would look at it every night and think about it.
And when it was dark and his eyes were closed, he could
   still see it.
And it was all of him.
And he loved it.
When he started school he brought it with him.
Not to show to anyone but just to have it with him,
   like a friend.
It was funny about school.
He sat in a square, brown desk
   like all other square, brown desks
   and he thought it should be red.
And his room was a square, brown room,
   like all the other rooms.
And it was tight and close.
And stiff.
He hated to hold the pencil and chalk,
   with his arm stiff and his feet flat on the floor,
   stiff, with the teacher watching and watching.
The teacher came and spoke to him.
She told him to wear a tie like all the other boys.
He said he didn't like them.
And she said it didn't matter!
After that they drew.
And he drew all yellow and it was the way he felt about
   morning.
And it was beautiful.
The teacher came and smiled at him.
"What's this?" she said. "Why don't you draw something like
   Ken's drawing? Isn't that beautiful?"
After that his mother bought him a tie.

And he always drew airplanes and rocket ships like everyone else.
And he threw the old picture away.
And when he lay alone looking at the sky,
   it was big and blue and all of everything,
   but he wasn't anymore.
He was square inside.
And brown.
And his hands were stiff.
And he was like everyone else.
And the things inside him that needed saying didn't need it anymore.
It had stopped pushing.
It was crushed.
Stiff.
Like everything else.

(This was written by a high school senior two weeks before he committed suicide.)

APPENDICES

RELIABILITY STUDY

RESULTS

THE raw scores in Tables 3 and 4 were statistically analyzed by Doctor Gary Lord, program evaluator, Department of Mental Health Sciences, Hahnemann Medical College and Hospital.

The Pearson Product Moment Correlation demonstrated a moderately significant correlation between rater 1 and the author ($r_1 = 0.69$, $p < 0.01$); a moderately significant correlation between rater 2 and the author ($r_2 = 0.43$, $p < 0.01$) and a lower, but still significant correlation between rater 1 and 2 ($r_{12} = 0.36$, $p < 0.05$) (see Table 5).

An intraclass test (based on one-way ANOVA, Guilford, 1965) was performed to determine typical reliability for the average of several raters (r_{kk}) and typical reliability for a single rater (r_{cc}). The results indicated that $r_{kk} = 0.73$ and, therefore, while not exceedingly high, the measure can be termed reliable. The result $r_{cc} = 0.48$ suggests that the measure is more reliable when used with more than one rater (see Table 6).

Doctor Lord also examined whether or not the three raters see about the same number of defenses and correlated the totals from the raw data. For rater 1 and the author, $r_{1A} = 0.29$ and is not significant; $r_{2A} = 0.39$, $p < 0.01$; $r_{12} = 0.02$ and is not significant.

Finally, the percentage of responses of each rater compared to the author was computed and the results are as follows: $r_1 = 62.02\%$, $r_2 = 17.76\%$.

DISCUSSION

In reviewing the results the reader must keep in mind that the measure (criteria for identifying manifestations of defense mechanisms in graphic productions, p. 129) proposed in this dissertation was not in fact the measure used by raters 1 and 2. The intent of having two raters respond to the same random sample of illustrations was to test the author's original contention that psychoanalytically trained

TABLE 3

Defense Mechanisms of the Ego Identified in a Random Sample of Drawings by Two Blind Raters and Correlated With Those Identified by the Author in Those Same Drawings*

Fig. #	Rater #1	Author	Rater #2
25A	projection, regression, repression, incorporation, undoing	projection, undoing (reversal), regression (incorporation), repression	denial, reversal, avoidance, regression, introjection
27A	undoing, denial, projection, regression, repression	identification, denial, repression, regression (incorporation), isolation of affect, projection	sublimation, regression, isolation
15C	isolation, projection, regression, repression	regression (incorporation), isolation of affect, projection	sublimation, regression, isolation
15A	projection, regression, repression, incorporation, isolation, undoing, denial	projection, reversal, avoidance, denial, sublimation, reaction-formation	isolation, sublimation, introjection
48C	projection, regression, repression, isolation, undoing, incorporation	projection, isolation, regression (incorporation) repression	introjection, isolation, identification, sublimation
48A	projection, regression, repression, incorporation	projection, imitation, early identification, repression	introjection
46C	projection, regression, repression, isolation, undoing, denial	repression, projection, denial, avoidance, isolation	undoing, turning against self, isolation
17B	projection, regression, undoing, repression	projection, regression (incorporation), isolation of affect	regression
16D	projection, regression, repression, isolation, undoing, denial	projection, reaction-formation, regression (incorporation)	intellectualization, regression, introjection

*Total Number of Possible Choices = 19

TABLE 3 (Continued)

Fig. #	Rater #1	Author	Rater #2
41C	projection, repression, regression, undoing, incorporation	projection, denial , isolation, regression (incorporation) undoing, reversal	undoing, turning against self, regression, incorporation
40B	projection, repression, regression, incorporation, denial	projection, regression (incorporation)	incorporation, regression
39	projection, repression, regression, denial	projection, denial, isolation	isolation
38C	projection, repression, regression, denial, isolation	projection, denial, avoidance, imitation, identification,	identification, identification with aggressor, denial, isolation
37C	projection, repression, regression, undoing, incorporation, denial	projection, repression, isolation of affect, reversal, rationalization	sublimation, displacement
31B	projection, regression, repression, incorporation, denial	projection, repression, isolation of affect, denial, identification	undoing, denial, regression, introjection
*	projection, regression, repression, undoing, denial	projection, repression, regression (incorporation), denial, reversal, undoing	regression, turning against self
*	projection, regression, repression, isolation, incorporation	projection, repression, denial, displacement	sublimation, introjection

*Frontispiece

TABLE 3 (Continued)

Fig. #	Rater #1	Author	Rater #2
*	isolation, incorporation, undoing denial, projection, regression, repression	projection, repression, isolation, denial, introjection	regression, introjection, turning against self
29	projection, repression, regression, isolation, incorporation, undoing	projection, repression, undoing (reversal), regression (incorporation)	isolation, avoidance, sublimation, introjection
15A	projection, repression, regression, isolation, undoing, denial	projection, avoidance, reversal, denial, identification, sublimation, reaction-formation	introjection, isolation sublimation
44A	projection, regression, repression, isolation, incorporation	projection, repression, isolation, denial, reversal, avoidance	avoidance, isolation, intellectualization, identification, introjection
46A	projection, regression, repression, isolation, incorporation, undoing	repression, projection, denial, avoidance	regression, avoidance
28A	projection, regression, repression, incorporation, undoing, denial	projection, repression, identification, isolation of affect, regression (incorporation)	displacement, sublimation
26A	projection, regression, repression, incorporation, intellectualization	projection, repression, denial, undoing/reversal, avoidance, isolation of affect	regression, isolation
24A	projection, regression, repression, undoing, denial, intellectualization	projection, repression, regression, undoing (incorporation)	intellectualization, displacement

*Frontispiece

TABLE 3 (Continued)

Fig. #	Rater #1	Author	Rater #2
16B	projection, regression, repression, isolation, incorporation, undoing	projection, reversal, displacement	intellectualization, regression, introjection
45A	projection, regression, repression, isolation, incorporation, intellectualization	projection, repression, regression (incorporation), denial, isolation, displacement	isolation, regression, intellectualization
37A	projection, regression, repression, denial, identification	projection, repression, identification, reversal, reaction-formation, regression (incorporation)	identification, displacement, reaction-formation, sublimation
36B	projection, regression, repression, isolation, incorporation, undoing	projection, repression, identification with aggressor, regression(incorporation), undoing (reversal), denial	avoidance, regression, reversal, introjection
36D	projection, repression, regression, incorporation	projection, repression, isolation, undoing, avoidance	introjection, isolation, regression, intellectualization
35B	projection, regression, repression, incorporation, undoing	projection, regression (incorporation), imitation, isolation, undoing, avoidance	isolation, regression, denial
14A	projection, regression, repression, undoing, isolation, denial	projection, denial, avoidance, undoing (reversal)	identification, reversal, displacement, sublimation
13B	projection, regression, repression, undoing, denial	projection, undoing	displacement

TABLE 3 (Continued)

Fig. #	Rater #1	Author	Rater #2
9	projection, regression, repression, undoing	projection, regression, incorporation	regression
22A	projection, regression, repression, undoing, denial, reaction-formation, intellectualization	projection, repression, denial, avoidance, isolation of affect	sublimation
21A	projection, regression, repression, isolation, intellectualization	projection, regression, isolation of affect, denial	regression, sublimation
19B	projection, regression, repression, isolation, undoing	projection, denial, isolation of affect	isolation, undoing, avoidance
18A	projection, regression, repression, isolation, incorporation, denial, reaction-formation	projection, isolation of affect, avoidance	isolation, undoing
43A	projection, regression, repression, undoing	projection, regression, isolation of affect, undoing, regression (incorporation)	regression, turned against self, intellectualization
42B	projection, regression, repression, denial, incorporation, undoing, intellectualization	projection, repression, identification with aggressor, isolation, denial, regression (incorporation)	denial, reversal
41E	projection, regression, repression	projection, repression, denial, reversal	turning against self, isolation, reversal, identification

TABLE 3 (Continued)

Fig. #	Rater #1	Author	Rater #2
23A	projection, regression, repression, undoing, intellectualization	projection, repression, denial	isolation, displacement
33B	projection, regression, repression, isolation, undoing, denial	projection, repression, displacement, isolation, sublimation, identification	intellectualization, avoidance, denial
32B	projection, regression, repression, isolation, undoing, denial	projection, repression, isolation of affect, denial, identification, identification with aggressor, regression (incorporation)	identification, intellectualization
34D	projection, regression, repression, incorporation, undoing, denial	projection, repression, avoidance, undoing (reversal), regression (incorporation), identification with aggressor	avoidance, turning against the self
34B	projection, repression, regression, isolation, incorporation, denial	projection, repression, isolation, identification, avoidance, regression (incorporation), imitation	regression, introjection, denial, reversal, turning against the self

TABLE 4

Number of Defense Mechanisms Identified by Author and 2 Raters; Number Raters were in Agreement With Author; Number They Omitted; Number They Added

Fig.	Rater #1				Rater #2				Author
	Total	Agreed	Omitted	Added	Total	Agreed	Omitted	Added	Total #
25A	5	5	1	0	5	2	3	3	6
27A	5	4	3	1	3	2	5	1	7
15C	4	3	2	1	3	2	2	1	5
15A	7	2	5	5	3	1	6	2	7
48C	6	5	0	1	4	1	4	3	5
48A	4	2	2	2	1	0	4	0	4
46C	6	4	1	2	3	1	4	2	5
17B	4	2	2	2	1	1	3	0	4
16D	6	2	2	4	3	1	3	2	4
41C	5	4	3	1	4	3	4	1	7
40B	5	4	1	0	2	2	3	0	5
39	4	3	0	1	1	1	2	0	3
38C	5	3	2	2	4	2	4	2	5
39C	6	2	3	4	2	0	5	2	5
31B	5	3	2	2	4	1	4	3	5
30B	5	5	2	0	2	1	5	1	7
*	5	2	2	3	2	0	4	2	4
*	7	4	1	3	3	1	4	2	5
29	6	5	1	1	4	0	6	4	6

*Frontispiece

TABLE 4 (Continued)

Fig.	Rater #1				Rater #2				Author
	Total	Agreed	Omitted	Added	Total	Agreed	Omitted	Added	Total #
15A	6	2	5	4	3	1	4	2	7
44A	5	3	3	2	5	2	4	3	6
46A	6	2	2	4	2	1	3	1	4
28A	6	4	2	2	2	0	6	2	6
26A	5	2	5	3	2	1	5	1	7
24A	6	4	1	2	2	0	5	2	5
16B	6	1	2	5	3	0	3	3	3
45A	6	5	2	1	3	2	4	1	7
37A	5	4	3	1	4	2	5	2	7
36B	6	5	3	1	4	2	6	2	8
36D	4	2	3	2	4	1	4	3	5
35B	5	4	3	1	3	2	5	1	7
14A	6	3	2	3	4	0	5	4	5
13B	5	2	0	3	1	0	2	1	2
9	4	2	1	2	1	1	2	0	3
22A	7	3	2	4	1	0	5	1	5
21A	5	3	1	2	2	0	4	2	4
19B	5	2	1	3	3	1	2	2	3
18A	7	2	1	5	2	1	2	1	3
43A	4	4	2	0	3	1	5	2	6

They Could Not Talk and So They Drew

TABLE 4 (Continued)

Fig.	Rater #1				Rater #2				Author
	Total	Agreed	Omitted	Added	Total	Agreed	Omitted	Added	Total#
42B	7	5	2	2	2	1	6	1	7
41E	3	2	2	1	4	1	3	3	4
23A	5	2	1	3	2	0	3	2	3
33B	6	3	3	3	3	0	6	3	6
32B	6	5	3	1	2	1	7	1	8
31D	6	5	3	1	2	1	7	1	8
34B	6	5	3	1	5	1	7	4	8

TABLE 5

Rater Responses Correlated With Author and Each Other Using
Pearson Product Moment Statistical Test

	r	t
Rater 1 & Author	0.69*	6.31
Rater 2 & Author	0.43*	3.20
Rater 1 & 2	0.36**	2.55

*p   0.01
**p   0.05

art therapists could identify a number of defense mechanisms in drawings.

Both raters received their graduate degrees from the Hahnemann program a number of years ago, but their experience since then has been quite different. Rater 1 graduated in 1972, has worked with a variety of populations, and in 1976 developed and directed a new graduate-training program in art therapy in a medical school in the South. Rater 2 graduated in 1977 and has worked primarily with retarded and severely disturbed populations. After the birth of her child two years ago, she retired from full-time employment, and her only involvement has been in a supervisory capacity for an art therapy intern working with disturbed children.

Rater 1 received no information about the individuals who produced the sample illustrations; rater 2 was given the age and the sex of each subject.

Given the conditions noted above, the results are greater than was expected. The high correlation between rater 1 and the author, in spite of no information, is attributed to his broader involvement in the field and continued use of the original training approach in the development of his own program. He appended his responses with a statement that he considered projection, regression and repression defenses present in all drawings. The author agrees with the former but believes developmental issues influence the presence of the latter two. This would also account for some of the differences in agreement.

TABLE 6

Intraclass r (based on a 1-way ANOVA)* k = 3; r = 46 (No. of Phenomena Examined by all 3 Raters

	r_{kk}	r_{cc}
Typical reliability for the average of several raters	0.73	
Typical reliability for a single rater		0.48

*Ref. Guilford, J.P.: Fundamental Statistics in Psychology of Education, 4th Ed. New York: McGraw-Hill, 1965, pp. 297-300.

Although rater 2 correlated significantly and she knew more about each subject, her limited involvement over the past years is seen as an important aspect of her lower correlation. Interestingly enough, another contributing factor is that she did have a significant correlation to the author in relation to the number of defenses identified. It is believed that having information pertaining to age and sex made her more conservative, where the absence of this information invited rater 1 to risk more responses.

The identification of the defense mechanism of "turning on the self" used by rater 2 is described in the literature as part of the process of reversal and is not described as a separate defense mechanism. Therefore, while identification of "turning on the self" may have the same meaning for rater 2 as "reversal" does for the author, it was counted in the "added" column and may account for some of the disagreement between the rater and the author.

CONCLUSION

The criteria for identifying adaptive and maladaptive defense mechanisms in drawings as proposed by the author have not been described elsewhere. This is a first attempt in this direction.

The results demonstrated by the analysis of the raters' responses hold considerable promise for future investigation. At this writing, a pilot study has been initiated by a current student of the author. Using the criteria developed, two groups of pre-school and first-grade emotionally disturbed children in a therapeutic center will be given pre- and post-evaluations over a six-month period. The investigator hypothesizes that the children whose mothers attend the parent group at the center will adapt better and perform better academically than those children whose mothers do not participate in the parent group. The measure developed here will be one of the instruments used. Regardless of the outcome, the results will have important implications for future studies.

It is also believed that training of investigators in this methodology will demonstrate greater reliability and that concurrent data from histories and available tests collected on subjects in future studies will provide validity for this measure.

TABLE 7

Comparison of Defenses Identified in Drawings by Author (A) and
Defenses Identified in Behavior by Psychologist/Psychiatrist (P)

Name_____ Age_____ Number of Drawings Reviewed_____

Spontaneous_____ Directed _____

Defenses	A	P	Agree
Incorporation			
Projection			
Displacement			
Isolation			
Rationalization			
Imitation			
Reversal			
Denial			
Undoing			
Identification			
Identification with Aggressor			
Regression			
Repression			

Author's note: Repression inherent in images produced after age 6-7
Incorporation seen in images indicating regression
Projection of "inner screen" seen in all images

(see TABLE 2 for further clarification)

Sample Scoring Sheet designed by Author for use by author, 1 Clinical
Psychologist/Music Therapist and 3 Psychoanalytically trained Child
Psychiatrists to rate 19 subjects ages 6 to 11 years of age.

Appendix B

VALIDITY STUDY

RESULTS

THE raw scores in Table 8 were statistically analyzed by Doctor Gary Lord, program evaluator, Department of Mental Health Sciences, Hahnemann University of Health Sciences.

The average percent of agreement between author (A) and psychologist or psychiatrist (P) of a possible 13 defense mechanisms of the ego (DEF) is 59.5 percent with a SD of 12.8 percent. This actually compares the number of DEF each child could possibly utilize at any time, with the number A identified in drawings and P identified in behavior, and provides no information on the validity of the author's criteria for DEF manifested in drawings.

Therefore, the percentage of agreement between A and P was calculated on the number of DEF present and absent for each subject. The average percent of agreement for DEF present was 70.8 percent with a SD of 15.1 percent and the average percent of agreement for DEF absent was 56.7 percent with a SD of 23.6 percent (see Table 9).

The Pearson Product Moment Correlation demonstrated no significant correlation of agreement on DEF present $-r = -0.14$, and absent $-r = -0.06$ (see Table 10).

The assumption was made that the presence or absence of each DEF was an independent variable, and a chi-square analysis was conducted. $C = 0.93$ and reveals no significant difference of agreement between A and P (see Table 11).

DISCUSSION

An effort was made to test the validity of the author's criteria for identifying defense mechanisms of the ego in spontaneous and or directed drawings of children. Three psychoanalytically trained child psychiatrists and one clinical psychologist, who is also a certified music therapist, all known to solicit drawings from their patients,

TABLE 8

Number and Percent of Agreement Between A and P on Total Possible Number
of Defense Mechanisms of the Ego. (Def.)

Subject	Age	No. of Agreements out of Possible 13 Def.	% Agreement
J	6	6	46
M	8.9	6	46
J	8	9	69
R	10,11	7	54
A	10	8	62
T	7.5	7	54
R	8	6	46
S	7	9	69
J	11	9	69
AB	10	10	71
ND	9	9	69
RB	7	9	69
X	9	8	62
TB	10	9	69
NA	8	9	69
GS	9	9	69
M	7	8	62
L	10	5	38
M	10.6	4	31

Average % agreement out of possible 13 DEF = 59.5%; SD 12.8%

This is a comparison of the number of DEF each child could possibly
utilize at any time with the number A identified in drawings and
P identified in behavior and provides no information on the
validity of the author's criteria for DEF manifested in drawings.

were asked to participate in this small study.

The population consisted of nineteen subjects, four from one
psychiatrist, three from each of the other two psychiatrists and nine
from the clinical psychologist. All but one of the children were being
treated for some form of neurosis. One child was ego disturbed
manifesting more emotional impairment than the others.

TABLE 9

Number and Per Cent Agreement of A with P of Defenses Present and
Defenses Absent

Subject	Age	No. of Defenses Present			No. of Defenses Absent		
		A	P	% Agreement	A	P	% Agreement
J	6	6	11	55	7	2	29
M	8.9	6	11	55	5	2	40
J	8	8	10	80	5	3	60
R	10,11	9	9	100	4	4	100
A	10	8	9	89	5	4	80
T	7.5	8	11	73	5	1	20
R	8	8	9	89	5	4	80
S	7	8	12	67	5	1	20
J	11	7	11	63	6	2	33
AB	10	5	4	80	8	9	88
ND	9	9	6	67	4	7	57
RB	7	8	6	75	5	7	71
X	9	8	3	37.5	5	10	50
TB	10	11	7	64	2	6	33
NA	8	9	7	78	4	6	67
GS	9	10	6	60	3	7	43
M	7	8	9	89	5	4	80
L	10	5	8	62.5	8	5	63
M	10.6	5	8	62.5	8	5	63

Average % Agreement # of Defenses Present = 70.8%; S.D. −15.1%.
Average % Agreement of Defenses Absent = 56.7%; S.D. 23.6%

The results indicate a better than chance % agreement.

The author discussed nineteen DEF on a hierarchical scale in the text of this work. Only thirteen DEF were selected for this study and are listed in Table 7. The decision to omit six of the nineteen DEF was made by the author, in consultation with Mrs. Janet Hoopes, Ph.D., chairman, Department of Child Development and Education, Bryn Mawr College, and was based on the facts that some defenses could not be identified in drawings without associations (see Table 2), and the other participating clinicians had no familiarity

TABLE 10

A & P Responses of # Present and # Absent Correlated Using Pearson
Product Moment Statistical Test

	P	t_t
Present A c̄ P	−.14	−.57
Absent A c̄ P	−.06	−.26

The results indicate there is no significant correlation between
A and P.

with the chronological order and criteria developed by the author.

The psychologist, psychiatrists and the author rated the children
and drawings separately and the results were compared and analyzed. The author rated fifty-one drawings; seven for each of two
subjects and only one for one subject. The clinical psychologist informed the author that the drawings she provided were done over a
three-year period, and she could not correlate the time the drawings
were done with the times certain DEF were observed in behavior.
There was no information on the relationship of observation of
behavior and when the drawings were done from the psychiatrists.

While the results indicate that there is no significant correlation
they also demonstrate there is no significant difference in agreement
between A and P. The average percent of agreement, 70.8 percent,
also suggests further research might demonstrate a higher degree of
correlation. The analysis of the data reveals that the author, in many
cases, saw more defenses in drawings than the more traditional clinicians saw in behavior. This was expected by the author, who
believes that spontaneous drawings often reveal more than observations of behavior. This, plus the difference in training of art therapists versus traditional clinical psychologists and psychoanalysts,
could well account for the low correlation of this limited study. It
should also be noted that there are no studies that validate criteria
used by psychoanalysts to observe defenses in behavior.

TABLE 11

Chi Square Contingency Table
  Assumption: Presence and absence of Each Defense was Independent Variable

	PRESENT	ABSENT	
A	146 (151.2)	157 (151.8)	303
P	99 (193.8)	89 (94.2)	188
	245	246	491

$$c = \sqrt{\frac{.93}{491 + .93}} = .04$$

The results indicate there is no significant difference of
agreement between A and P.

While the scope of this work did not allow for a discussion of the relationship of spontaneous drawings to standardized projective techniques, a comparison of these two measures would be useful in providing validation data. In discussion with Doctor Herman Belmont, deputy chairman, Department of Mental Health Sciences, Hahnemann University, it was noted that the Rorschach test and the TAT often identify more defenses than an initial clinical interview.

CONCLUSION

The results point to a better-than-chance agreement between A and P and suggest strong implications for further study of validity. To do so, one possibility would be a larger population including only normal children, randomly selected, who would be administered the Rorschach, the TAT and requested to do at least three spontaneous drawings. The results of these three measures could be analyzed in a variety of ways. Another possibility would be to use these same measures, plus psychiatrists' observations of a patient population. In this case, the participating psychiatrists would be cognizant of the author's theoretical construct and basis for identifying criteria of DEF in drawings. This collection of data has infinite possibilities for statistical analysis. Further study is necessary before the measure for identifying defenses in drawings as proposed by the author can either be rejected or fully accepted as valid.

GLOSSARY OF PIAGETIAN TERMS

ACCOMMODATION: One of the two aspects of adaptation in which the cognitive structure is modified to conform with the contours of external reality. It is progressive in nature as it involves change, although it is always accompanied by assimilation, which is conservative.

ADAPTATION: A biological activity of all life in which, at the simplest level, there is preservation and survival. Piaget, however, emphasizes adaptation as a process in which the organism, through interaction with the environment, is transformed in such a way that its preservation is enhanced. Hence, there occurs a shift from less stable to more stable equilibrium. In adaptation, assimilation and accommodation function in a complementary fashion moving the organism toward progressive equilibrium. It is the one of the two functional invariants which deal with the external aspect of development.

AFFECT: The behavioral component which deals with motivation, energy, interest, and values. It is indissociable from cognition. Psychic functioning is always characterized by both affect and cognition.

ANIMISM: A characteristic of the pre-operational mind in which inanimate objects in the external world are viewed by the child as possessing human attributes such as will, life, volitional force, and a capacity for feeling.

ARTIFICIALISM: Refers to the pre-operational child's belief that natural objects in the world, such as mountains and the stars, were made by men for human purposes. For example, the child may express the belief, when questioned, that the stars were made and placed in the sky by his father for the purpose of providing us with a way of seeing outdoors at nighttime.

ASSIMILATION: One of the two aspects of adaptation in which external reality is incorporated into existing cognitive structures. It

Reprinted by permission from Hugh Rosen, Ph.D.

is conservative in nature as it does not involve change, although it is always accompanied by accommodation, which is progressive.

CENTRATION: Involves focusing on one aspect of a phenomenon to the exclusion of other aspects. It may be perceptual, as in attending the height of a container of water while disregarding the width in a liquid conservation task, or it may be non-perceptual, as in focusing exclusively upon one's own point of view while failing to take into account another's viewpoint. The result is a distortion of the objective situation.

CIRCULAR REACTION: The infant's own actions by chance produce an unexpected effect, which then leads to a deliberate repetition of the act to reinstate the effect. Once the action has been carried out accidentally, the effect may continuously trigger it again throughout numerous cycles. The circular reaction develops through several sensorimotor stages progressing from stereotyped, body-centered activities toward novel and object-focused actions.

CONCRETE OPERATIONAL PERIOD: The third major period of cognitive development. Thinking is highly organized and systematic, derived from structural groupings of classification and seriation. The child of this period comprehends number and can conserve. His thinking is decentered, attends transformations, and is reversible. Logical thinking is confined, however, to concrete objects in the environment or to mental representations of familiar objects (7 to 11 years).

CONSERVATION: The cognitive competence, derived from a developed structure, to realize that despite certain modifications of an object some properties of the object remain unchanged. For example, the pre-operational child does not recognize that a clay ball elongated into a sausage shape will retain the same amount of substance or weight. The concrete operational child does know this, and his knowing is based upon having constructed structures of identity, compensation, and negation, which promote information processing of the observed data.

DECENTRATION: A cognitive activity in which multiple aspects of a phenomenon are taken into account. In a limited version this occurs sequentially, but at a more advanced level it occurs simultaneously. Simultaneous decentering facilitates the coordination of the various aspects and leads to objective knowledge.

EGOCENTRIC: Verbal communication in which the speaker is

unaware that the listener may have a different point of view and specific needs which must be met in order to comprehend the message. As a result, the speaker makes no attempt to prove his assertions or to meet the listener's informational needs. The speaker's syntax suffers accordingly.

EGOCENTRISM: A cognitive incapacity to differentiate between subjective and objective components. The person is embedded in his own perspective and lacks the capacity to adopt alternate viewpoints. Each period of development overcomes the form of egocentrism specific to it, but the newly emerging period is characterized by still another type of this limitation.

EPISTEMOLOGY: A study of the nature of knowledge and the manner in which it is acquired. Genetic epistemology is the field of study which approaches the acquisition of knowledge from a developmental standpoint.

EQUILIBRATION: A self-regulative mechanism accounting for stage transitions through progressive equilibrium. It involves a process in which external disturbances are compensated for by mental activity. In Piaget's terms, a more adaptive level of equilibrium is achieved by resolving cognitive conflicts which have induced a state of disequilibrium.

FIGURATIVE KNOWLEDGE: Refers to the static configuration of objects or events and stresses the sensorial component. The forms of cognition involved are perception, imitation, and mental images. An understanding of the figurative element by the individual is derived from his operative level of development. For example, figurative knowledge may entail a mental image of a human body. Understanding that representation in terms of anatomical and physiological systems, however, would require a fairly high level of operative development. Figurative and operative knowledge constitute two aspects of cognition through which something can be known and, hence, are not mutually exclusive.

FORMAL OPERATIONAL PERIOD: The fourth major period of cognitive development. Reality becomes a subset of the total range of possibilities. The adolescent thinker is capable of combinatorial analysis and hypothetico-deductive thought. Implementation of the scientific methodology is within the conceptual powers of the formal operational thinker. Reasoning can be dissociated from actual content and can be applied to the relationship between propositions

(11 years onward).

FUNCTIONAL INVARIANTS: Comprised of adaptation and organization. They are so called because these interrelated processes continue to function in the same manner, without qualitative change, throughout all cognitive development and mental activity. In contrast, cognitive structures undergo qualitative change over the course of development.

IRREVERSIBILITY: A cognitive inability to follow a process from beginning to end and then retrace the steps back to the starting point. The lack of reversible thinking subjects the child to contradictory and unsystematic thought processes.

OPERATION: An internalized mental action characterized by the property of reversibility. Operations do not function in isolation but as integral parts of a complex structural network. Operations consist of such mental actions as combining, subtracting, multiplying, dividing, equal to, greater than, less than, etc. These mental actions are always performed and understood in relation to the total cognitive system. Cognitive acts of the pre-operational period, in contradistinction, are executed in isolation and not grasped in relation to a structural system.

OPERATIVE: Involves an act of transformation through which incoming data is understood. Its scope extends throughout all periods of cognitive development, and it should not be confused with the term *operational*, which refers only to the last two major periods of cognitive development. The meaning imposed upon the figurative element is derived from the particular level of operative development. The sensory input which constitutes figurative knowing is subject to a transformation determined by the operative or structural level of the knower (see Figurative Knowledge).

ORGANIZATION: A biological property of life in which the parts of an organism are related to one another and to the whole. At the most primitive level, an example would be the coordination of visual and grasping schemes into a more complex scheme of "grasping to look." An example at a more mature level of cognitive functioning would be the integration of classification and seriation structures to produce an understanding of number. It is the one of the two functional invariants which deals with the internal aspect of development.

PARTICIPATION: A pre-operational characteristic of mind in which the child assumes some causal connections between his own actions and things in the real world when these are, in fact, nonexistent. He may, for example, state that his own walking along a road causes the moon to follow his movements in the sky.

PRE-OPERATIONAL PERIOD: The second major period of cognitive development. Characterized by an advance to representation but limited by centrating, static, and irreversible thought. The child's world view is marked by features of animism, realism, artificialism, and participation. The pre-operational child does not conserve, and his thinking is not part of a systematic network of organized structures (2 to 7 years).

REALISM: A characteristic of the pre-operational mind in which a psychic phenomenon is accorded external, substantial existence by the child. For example, such purely psychic events as dreams and names are viewed by the child as existing independently in the physical world. There is a confusion on the child's part between his own thought and the nature of real objects in the world.

REVERSIBILITY: A cornerstone of intelligence first appearing in the logical operations of the concrete operational period. Involves the mental capacity to carry out an action in both directions. There are two types: inversion or negation $(A + B = C$, hence $C - B = A)$ and reciprocity $(A = B$, hence $B = A)$.

ROLE-TAKING: An ability to see perspectives other than one's own. Commonly referred to as putting yourself in the other person's shoes. It involves decentering so that the individual no longer focuses exclusively on his own point of view.

SCHEME: An internal cognitive structure of the sensorimotor period which is the source of a class of action sequences performed by the infant. For example, the infant engages in a number of varying specific acts of grasping. Together they constitute a class of acts which, although they differ in their specific features, all derive from a general cognitive structure known as a *grasping scheme*. Hence, a scheme designates an organized pattern of behavior. In a broad sense, it may refer to a governing plan of action at any level of development.

SEMIOTIC FUNCTION: Marks the beginning of symbolic or representational thought at approximately eighteen months. It is comprised of signs and symbols. Signs are public and arbitrary, such as words and symbols of the kind used in mathematics and science. Symbols are motivated and private as in dreams, images, symbolic play and deferred imitation. In his earlier work, Piaget referred to the semiotic function as the symbolic function.

SENSORIMOTOR PERIOD: The first major period of cognitive development. During this time, the infant progresses from pure reflex activity to symbolic functioning. He constructs a knowledge of reality on a behavioral plane in dimensions of space, time, causality, intentionality, and object permanence (0 to 2 years).

SIGNIFIER: A sign or symbol which represents an object not present to the perceptual apparatus. The represented object is referred to as the signified. The meaning assigned to the representation is known as the significate.

SOCIOCENTRIC: Verbal communication which is adapted to the listener's informational needs. The speaker is aware that the other may have another point of view and he is able to see things from the listener's perspective.

TRANSDUCTION: An early pre-operational mode of reasoning in which the child goes from particular to particular in a process that links together elements that have no genuine causal or logical connection. It is neither inductive nor deductive. It exists largely becaue the child lacks cognitive structures that promote his understanding of classification and relations. Hence, it is most prevalent during the pre-conceptual phase of the pre-operational period.

BIBLIOGRAPHY

Alshuler, R.H., and Hattwick, L.B.W.: *Painting And Personality*. Chicago: The University of Chicago Press, 1947 (rev. ed. 1969).

Anthony, E.J.: Six applications de la théorie génétique de Piaget à la théorie et a la pratique de la psychodynamique. *Schweizerische Zielschrift Med Psychol, 29*, 20-34, 1956.

Arnheim, R.: *Art and Visual Perception*. Berkeley: University of California Press, 1954 (rev. ed. 1974).

Arnheim, R.: *Visual Thinking*. Berkeley: University of California Press, 1969.

Blatt, S.J.; Allison, J.; and Baker, B.L.: The Wechsler object assembly subtest and bodily concern. *Journal Consult Clin Psychol, 29*:223-230, 1965.

Bruner, J.S.: The course of cognitive growth. *American Psychologist, 19*:1-15, 1964.

Cobliner, W.G.: Psychoanalysis and the Geneva school of genetic psychology: parallels and counterparts. *International Journal of Psychiatry, 3*:82-129, 1967.

Coles, R.: *Erik Erikson, The Growth of His Work*. Boston: Little Brown, 1970.

Dabrowski, K.: Foreword. In Piechowski, M.M.: A theoretical and empirical approach to the study of development. *Genetic Psychology Monograph, 92*:233-237, 1975.

Decarie, T. Goyin: *Intelligence and Affectivity in Early Childhood*. New York: International Universities Press, 1965.

DiLeo, J.H.: *Children's Drawings as Diagnostic Aids*. New York: Bruner-Mazel, 1973.

Fink, P.J.: Art as a language. *Journal of Albert Einstein Medical Center, 15*:143-150, 1967.

Fink, P.J.: Art as a reflection of mental status. *Art Psychotherapy, 1*(1):17-30, 1973.

Fink, P.J.; Goldman, M.J.; and Levick, M.F.: Art therapy, a new discipline. *Pennsylvania Medicine, 70*:60-66, 1967.

Flavell, J.H.: Stage related properties of cognitive development. *Cognitive Psychology, 2*, 421-453, 1971.

Forisha, B.D.: Mental imagery verbal processes: a developmental study. *Developmental Psychology, 11* (3), 259-267, 1975.

Freud, A.: *The Ego and the Mechanisms of Defense*, rev. ed. New York: International Universities Press, 1966.

Freud, A.: Normality and pathology in childhood: assessments of development. In *The Writings of Anna Freud*. New York: International Universities Press, 1965, vol. VI.

Freud, S.: *An Outline of Psychoanalysis*. The James Strachey Translation. New York: W.W. Norton & Co., Inc., 1969.

Furth, H.G.: *Thinking Without Language*. Englewood Cliffs, N.J.: Prentice-Hall, 1966.

197

Galin, D.: Implications for psychiatry of left- and right-brain cerebral specialization. *Archives General Psychiatry, 31*:572-583, 1974.

Gantt, L., and Strauss, M.: *Art Therapy — A Bibliography, January 1940–June 1973.* National Institute of Mental Health, 1974.

Gardner, H.: *The Arts and Human Development.* New York: John Wiley and Sons, 1973.

Gardner, H.: *Artful Scribbles — The Significance of Children's Drawings.* New York: Basic Books, Inc., 1980.

Goodenough, F.L.: *Measurement of Intelligence by Drawings.* Yonkers-on-Hudson, New York: World Book Co., 1926.

Goodenough, F.L.: Studies in the psychology of children's drawings. *Psych Bull, 25*:272-283, 1928.

Greenspan, S.I.: Intelligence and adaptation. In Schlesinger, H.J. (Ed.): *Psychological Issues.* New York: International Universities Press, Inc., 1979.

Haber, R.N.: Where are the visions in visual perception? In Segal, S.J. (Ed.): *Imagery — Current Cognitive Approaches.* New York: Academic Press, 1971, pp. 36-48.

Hammer, E.F.: *The Clinical Application of Projective Drawing,* 2nd ed. Springfield: Thomas, 1978.

Hardiman, G.W., and Zernich, T.: Some considerations of Piaget's cognitive-structuralist theory and children's artistic development. *Studies In Art Education, 23*:3, 1980.

Harms, E.: The development of modern art therapy. *Leonardo, 8*:241-244, 1975.

Hartman, H.: *Ego Psychology and the Problem of Adaptation.* New York: International Universities Press, 1958.

Hatterer, L.J.: *The Artist in Society.* New York: Grove Press, 1965.

Holt, R.R.: The development of the primary process: a structural view. In Holt, R.R. (Ed.): *Motives and Thought Psychoanalytic Essays in Honor of David Rappaport* (Psychological Issues, Monograph). New York: International Universities Press, 1967, pp. 345-383.

Horowitz, M.J.: *Image Formation and Cognition.* New York: Appleton-Century-Crofts, 1970.

Inhelder, B., and Piaget, J.: *The Growth of Logical Thinking from Childhood to Adolescence.* Translated by A. Parsons and S. Milgram. New York: Basic Books, 1958 (originally published, 1955).

Kaplan, L.: Object constancy in the light of Piaget's vertical décalage. *Bulletin Menninger Clinic, 36*:322-334, 1972.

Kellogg, R. with O'Dell, S.: *The Psychology of Children's Art.* New York: CRM — Random House Publication, 1967.

Kellogg, R.: *Analyzing Children's Art.* Palo Alto, California: Mayfield Publishing Co., 1969, 1970.

Kestenberg, J.S.: *Children and Parents: Psychoanalytic Studies in Development.* New York: Jason Aronson, 1975.

Kolb, L.C.: *A Psychiatric Glossary.* Washington, D.C.: American Psychiatric Assoc., 1969.

Koppitz, E.M.: *Psychological Evaluation of Children's Human Figure Drawings.* New York:

Grune and Stratton, 1968.

Kramer, E.: Art therapy at Wiltwyck school. *School Arts, 58*:5-8, 1958*a*.

Kramer, E.: *Art Therapy in a Children's Community*. Springfield: Thomas, 1958*b*.

Kris, E.: *Psychoanalytic Explorations in Art*. New York: International Universities Press, 1952.

Kubie, L.S.: *Neurotic Distortion of the Creative Process*. Lawrence, Kansas: University of Kansas Press, 1958.

Kwiatkowska, H.: The use of families' art productions in psychiatric evaluation. *Bulletin of Art Therapy, 6*:52-69, 1967. (with discussion by N.L. Paul, pp. 69-72)

Kwiatkowska, H.: *Family Therapy and Evaluation Through Art*. Springfield: Thomas, 1978.

Levick, M.F.; Goldman, M.J.; and Fink, P.J.: Training for art therapists: community mental health center and college of art join forces. *Bulletin of Art Therapy, 6*:121-124, 1967.

Levick, M.F.: The goals of the art therapist as compared to those of the art teacher. *Journal of Albert Einstein Medical Center, 15*:157-170, 1967.

Levick, M.F.: Family art therapy in the community. *Philadelphia Medicine, 69*:257-261, 1973.

Levick, M.F., and Herring, J.: Family dynamics — as seen through art therapy. *Art Psychotherapy, 1*:45-54, 1973.

Levick, M.F.: Transference and countertransference as manifested in graphic productions. *International Journal of Art Psychotherapy* (U.S.A.), *2*:203-224, 1975.

Levick, M.F.; Dulicai, D.; Briggs, C.; and Billock, I.: The creative arts therapies. In Adamson, William, and Adamson, K. (Eds.): *A Handbook for Specific Learning Disabilities*. New York: Gardner Press, 1979.

Levick, M.F.; Donnelly, G.; and Snyder, S.: A Study of the Relationship Between Cognitive and Psychosexual Development. Unpublished Paper, Bryn Mawr, 1979.

Levick, M.F.: Art therapy: an overview. In Corsini, R. (Ed.): *Handbook of Innovative Psychotherapies*. New York: John Wiley & Sons, 1981, pp. 51-68.

Lewis, M.M.: *Language, Thought, and Personality*. New York: Basic Books, 1963.

Lowenfeld, V.: *The Nature of Creative Activity*. In Alschuler, R., and Hattwick, L.W.: *Painting and Personality*. Chicago and London: The University of Chicago Press, 1969, p. 118.

Machover, K.: *Personality Projection in the Drawing of the Human Figure*, 2nd ed. Springfield: Thomas, 1978.

Mahler, M.S.: *On Human Symbiosis and the Vicissitudes of Individuation*. New York: International Universities Press, 1968.

Mahler, M.; Pine, F.; and Bergman, A.: *The Psychological Birth of the Human Infant*. New York: Basic Books, 1975.

Moore, B.E., and Fine, B.D. (Eds.): *A Glossary of Psychoanalytic Terms and Concepts*, 2nd ed. New York: The American Psychoanalytic Association, 1968.

Nagera, H.: *Vincent van Gogh: A Psychological Study*. New York: International Universities Press, 1967.

Naumburg, M.: *Studies of Free Art Expression in Behavior of Children as a Means of Diagnosis and Therapy*. New York: Coolidge Foundation, 1947.

Naumburg, M.: *Dynamically Oriented Art Therapy: Its Principals and Practice*. New York: Grune and Stratton, 1966.

Neale, J.M.: Egocentrism in institutionalized and noninstitutionalized children. *Child Development, 37*:97-101, 1966.

Noy, P.: The psychoanalytic theory of cognitive development. In Solnit, J.; Eissler, R.; Freud, A.; Kris, M.; and Neubauer, P. (Eds.): *The Psychoanalytic Study of the Child*. New Haven: Yale Universities Press, 1979.

Odier, C.: *Anxiety and Magical Thinking*. New York: International Universities Press, 1956.

Paivio, A.: Imagery and language. In Segal, S.J. (Ed.): *Imagery — Current Cognitive Approaches*. New York: Academic Press, 1971, pp. 9-30.

Piaget, J.: *Play, Dreams, and Imitation in Childhood*. Translated by C. Gattegno and F.M. Hodgson. New York: W.W. Norton, 1962 (originally published, 1946).

Piechowski, M.M.: A theoretical and empirical approach to the study of development. *Genetic Psychology Monographs, 92*:231-297, 1975.

Rappaport, D.: The autonomy of the ego. In Knight, R.P., and Friedman, C.R. (Eds.): *Psychoanalytic Psychiatry and Psychology*. New York: International Universities Press, 1954.

Rappaport, D.: *Psychoanalytic Psychiatry and Psychology*. In Greenspan, S.I.: *Intelligence and Adaptation*. New York: International Universities Press, Inc., 1979, p. 255.

Rosen, H.: *Pathway to Piaget*. Cherry Hill, New Jersey: Postgraduate International, 1977.

Rothgeb, C.L. (Eds.): *Abstracts of the Standard Edition of Freud*. Washington, D.C.: Department of Health, Education, and Welfare, 1971/2.

Selman, R.L.: Social cognitive understanding: A guide to educational and clinical practice. In Lickona, T. (Ed.): *Moral Development and Behavior*. New York: Holt, Rinehart and Winston, 1976, pp. 299-316.

Stern, M.: Free Paint as an Auxiliary Technique in Psychotherapy. In Bychowski, G., and Despert, L. (Eds.): *Specialized Techniques in Psychotherapy*. New York: Basic Books, 1952.

Ulman, E.: Art therapy: Problems of definition. *Bulletin of Art Therapy, 1*:10-20, 1961.

Ulman, E.: Therapy is not enough — the contribution of art to general hospital psychiatry. *Bulletin of Art Therapy, 6*:13-21, 1966.

Vaccaro, V.M.: Specific aspects of the psychology of art therapy. *International Journal of Art Psychotherapy* (U.S.A.), *1*:81-89, 1973.

Vygotsky, L.S.: *Thought and Language*. Translated by E. Hanfmann and G. Vakar. Cambridge, Mass.: The MIT Press, 1962 (originally published, 1934).

Wolff, P.H.: The developmental psychologies of Jean Piaget and psychoanalysis. *Psychological Issues, Monograph*. New York: International Universities Press, 1960, vol. 5.

Zetzel, E.: The so-called good hysteric. In *The Capacity for Emotional Growth*. New York: International Universities Press, 1970, pp. 229-245.

Zwerling, I.: The creative arts as real therapies. *Hospital and Community Psychiatry, 30(12)*:841-844, 1979.

INDEX

A

Abnormal, ix, xix, 25, 147 (*see also specific mental disorders*)
Abuse, 145 (*see also* Sexual abuse, Trauma)
Accommodation, 35, 135, 191
Acting out, 148, 163
Activity, 145
Adaptation, 191
  cognitive, 75
  defenses in, xviii, 14, 20, 23, 28, 35, 39, 63, 65, 71, 77, 93, 94, 96, 128, 165, 182
    illustration of, *Fig. 32A & B* 110
  social, 12, 20, 21, 23, 33, 35, 161
Adjunctive therapy, 15
Adolescence, 25, 27, 134, 135
  upheaval in, 26, 100
Adolescents, xii, xv, 20, 25, 34, 35, 53, 106
Adulthood, xi, xii, xv, 25, 27, 57, 134
Adults, xx, 10, 14, 18, 22, 34, 46, 54, 163
Affect, xi, xii, 16, 19, 26, 30, 99, 101, 191
Age adequateness, 20 (*see also* Development, Developmental, Hierarchal developmental model of defense mechanisms)
Aggression, 72, 106, 143, 145
  illustration of, *Fig. 33A & B* 111
Aggressor (*see* Identification with aggressor)
Alcoholic patients, 13
Allison, J., 140
Alshuler, R. H., 79
Altruism, xxi, 26
Ambivilance, 104
American Art Therapy Association, 3, 5, 6, 7
American Journal of Art Therapy, 7
American Society for the Psychopathology of Expression, xix
Anal, xviii, 27, 59, 66, 86, 162 (*see also* Developmental sequences, Psychosexual development)

Analyses, 17
Anger, 9, 13, 143, 162
Animals, 45
Animism, 17, 23, 33, 65, 77, 135, 191
Annihilation, 140
Anthony, E. J., 40
Anxiety, 68, 89, 98, 102, 106, 113, 139, 143, 148
  castration, 17, 25, 139
  illustrations of, *Fig. 26A & B* 10, *Fig. 35E* 118
  objective of, 22
  object of, 63
  states, 19, 27, 28, 38
Arnheim, Rudolph, vii, 53, 55, 56, 60, 66, 80, 89, 161, 165
Art, 65 (*see also* Diagnosis, Therapeutic process)
  as a language, ix
  healing quality of, 8
  origins of, vii
Art education, 3, 56
Art media, viii, 10, 11, 12, 32, 39, 49, 65, 69, 70, 79, 102
  illustrations of, *Fig. 11* 71
Art product, 102
Art psychotherapy, xvii, 3, 5, 11, 137, 148
Art teachers, 59
Art therapists, 64, 106, 165
  role of, xv, xvii, 3, 5, 6, 7, 8, 12, 13, 39, 57, 88, 150
  training of, 38, 181, 188
Art therapy
  clinical application of, ix, xviii, 11-14, 164
  definition of, 3-4
  history of, 4-8
  methodology of, 5, 8, 10-11, 14, 142, 162
  sessions, 10, 142
  theory of, xv, xvii, 5, 8-10, 15, 35, 43, 56, 64, 157, 161

training in, 3, 6, 7, 8, 64
with children, 4, 10, 14
with families, 10, 11, 13, 14
with groups, 10
with individuals, 10, 14
Artificialism, 33, 77, 191
Artistic expression, viii, 44, 102, 120 (*see also* Drawings)
development of, ix, xv, 53, 60, 78, 80, 93, 99, 102, 105, 112, 162
illustrations of, *Fig. 12A* 73, *Fig. 13A & B* 74, *Fig. 16A* 84, *Fig. 34C* 115, Fig. 48A, B & C 160
illustration of, *Fig. 37A* 124
Assimilation, 35, 43, 71, 135, 191
Associations, 64, 78, 89, 102, 106, 143
Ault, Robert, 6
Autistic, 41
Avoidance, xxi, 22, 24, 25, 63, 65, 72, 75, 80, 87, 93, 99, 112, 113, 120, 127, 150, 152, 162
definition of, *Table 2* 131
illustrations of, *Fig. 14* 76, *Fig. 22A & B* 94, *Fig. 34A & B* 114, *Fig. 34D* 115, *Fig. 36E* 123, *Fig. 38C & D* 127
Awe, 80

B

Baker, B. L., 140
Balance, 20, 67, 88, 158
Baseline, 97, 109, 112, 139
illustrations of, *Fig. 42C* 147
Behavior, 126, 134 (*see also* Defense Mechanisms of the ego, Development)
adaptive, 38, 41, 43, 57, 59, 63
maladaptive, xxi, 35, 43, 59, 99, 106, 134, 140, 152
Behavioral psychology, xviii
Belmont, Herman, xxiii
Bergman, A., 23
Billock, Lisa, 14
Blatt, S. J., 140
Boszormenyi-Nagy, Ivan, 105
Boundaries, 135
ages related to, 64
between ego and superego, 96
external, 17, 18, 28, 42, 55, 59, 65, 140, 146
internal, 17, 18, 28, 42, 55, 59, 65, 140, 146

Brain damage, 142, 155, 165, (*see also* Organicity)
illustrations of, *Fig. 42A, B & C* 144, Fig. 47A, B & C 165
Briggs, Cynthia A., xxiii, 14
Bruner, Jerome S., 58
Buck, J., 45
Bulletin of Art Therapy, 5
Bychowski, G., 4

C

Case illustrations and studies
abnormal development, *Figs. 39-48* 138-160
normal development, *Figs. 9-38* 66-127
three and four years of age, *Figs. 9-14B* 66-76
five-seven years of age, *Figs. 15-24* 75-96
seven-eleven years of age, *Figs. 24-33* 97-111
Castration (*see* Anxiety)
Catharsis, 9
Centration, 95, 192
Character disorder, 148
Childhood, xi, xii, 17, 20, 21, 26, 31, 35, 36, 63, 65, 95, 135
Children, xx, 10, 13, 14, 22, 23, 35, 36, 42, 45, 46, 49, 55, 56, 57, 58, 59, 64, 77, 80, 83, 86, 97, 128, 158, 163
Chronological (*see* Development, Hierarchal development model of defense mechanisms)
Circles, 45, 46, 67, 95 (*see also* Shapes within shapes)
illustration of, *Fig. 4* 50
Circular reaction, 192
Classification, 34, 77
Cobliner, W. G., 40
Cognitive development, xii, 12 (*see also* Development)
Cohen, Felice, 6
Coles, Robert, 15
Color, 8, 67, 70, 71, 78, 86, 93, 98, 99, 112, 119, 158
Communication, 27, 28, 57, 58, 72, 104, 161
Complex (*see* Castration, Oedipal)
Conceptualization, 105
Concrete Operational Period, 27, 30, 33, 34, 41, 42, 59, 77, 88, 90, 94, 98, 104, 113, 120, 123, 139, 148, 163, 192

illustrations of, *Fig. 21* 92, *Fig. 37A* 124, Fig. 37C 125, *Fig. 38C & D* 127

Condensation, 8, 21, 22, 43, 89

Conflict-free sphere of ego (*see* Ego)

Conflictual areas of the psyche, 9, 11, 14, 54, 55, 59, 134

Conscious, xi, 9, 42, 78, 136 (*see also* Unconscious)

Conservation, 34, 77, 192

Constitutional factors, 26 (*see also* Genetic)

Control, 66, 70, 71, 113

illustration of, *Fig. 12A* 73

Coping styles, 102, 106 (*see also* Adaptive, Maladaptive, Defenses, Ego function)

Countertransference, 148

Creative arts in therapy, xvii, 15

Creative process, 120, 161 (*see also* Process)

Criteria for identifying defenses in drawings, *Table 2* 129-132

Cultural, 42, 45, 68, 78, 163 (*see also* Environment)

D

Dabrowski, K., ix, 36, 37, 38, 43, 59

Daydreams, 44 (*see also* Fantasy)

Death, 8, 38, 91

Decarrie, T. Goyin, 139

Decentration, 33, 192

Decompensation

illustration of, *Fig. 48A, B & C* 160

Defense mechanisms of the ego, vii, ix, xv, xvii, xviii, xix, 16, 18, 21, 23, 26, 34, 43, 44, 55, 60, 100, 106, 142, 162 (*see also specific defenses*, Hierarchal developmental model of defense mechanisms)

definitions of, *Table 2* 129-132

primitive, 66

illustrations of, *Fig. 40 A & B* 141, *Fig. 41A, B & C* 144

Demons, 17, 22, 161

Denial, xxi, 20, 21, 22, 24, 63, 65, 75, 77, 80, 81, 86, 88, 89, 96, 98, 100, 103, 104, 105, 106, 109, 112, 113, 119, 120, 125, 126, 127, 134, 136, 142, 143, 150, 152

definition of, *Table 2* 131

illustrations of, *Fig. 16C & D* 85, *Fig. 22A & B* 94, *Fig. 23A & B*, 95, *Fig. 27A & B & B* 101, *Fig. 30A & B* 107, *Fig. 31A & B* 107, *Fig. 35E* 118, *Fig. 36A* 121, *Fig. 36E* 123,

Fig. 37B 124, *Fig. 38A* 126, *Fig. 38C & D* 127, *Fig. 39* 138, *Fig. 41A, B & C* 144, *Fig. 42A* 146

Dependency, 72, 150

Depression, 4, 13, 38, 78, 162

Design, 49, 102, 112

Despert, L., 4

Development (*see also* Case illustrations and studies)

cognitive, vii, ix, xv, xix, xx, 16, 29, 30-35, 36, 41, 42, 43, 44, 53, 56, 59, 60, 63, 64, 66, 71, 72, 81, 86, 93, 102, 105, 113, 120, 134, 164

illustrations of, *Fig. 16A* 84, *Fig. 34C* 115, *Fig. 48A, B & C* 160

ego, xii, 12, 17, 18, 22, 26, 28, 98

emotional, ix, xix, 14, 38, 44, 59, 60, 71, 72, 81

motoric, 14, 32, 51, 102

illustrations of, *Fig. 8* 52, *Fig. 36B* 121

normal, xviii, 63-132

illustrations of, *Figs. 9-38* 66-127

perceptual, 14, 141, 143

illustration of, *Fig. 41D* 145

personality, xix, 3, 28, 30, 31, 134, 164, 165

psychosexual, vii, viii, xv, xx, 16, 29, 30, 32, 45, 56, 63, 64, 77, 79, 81, 86, 93, 105, 134, 164, 165

illustration of, *Fig. 37B* 124

Developmental (*see also* Developmental lines)

relationships, xv, 16, 28, 41, 42, 53, 56, 60, 134, 140

illustration of, *Figs. 40A & B* 141

sequences, 40, 45, 53, 59, 64, 113, 128, 134, 163

stages, xvii, xviii, 14, 23, 25, 28, 38, 53, 54, 59, 63, 65

Developmental lines (*see also* Case illustrations and studies)

correlation of cognitive, artistic, psychosexual and defenses, *Table 1* 61-62

illustrations of, *Fig. 37B* 124

Diagnosis (*see also* Case illustrations and studies)

art as, xviii, 4, 20, 24, 45, 165

DiLeo, J. H., ix, 53

Directed drawings, xvi, xx

Disharmony, 140 (*see also* Equilibrium)

illustrations of, *Fig. 40A & B* 141

Disorders (*see specific emotional/mental and organic disorders*)
Displacement, 8, 17, 21, 22, 25, 43, 63, 72, 80, 81, 91, 105, 106, 136, 145, 152, 158
definition of, *Table 2* 129
illustrations of, *Fig. 16B* 84, *Fig. 21* 92, *Fig. 32A & B* 110
Donnelly, Gloria, 45
Drawings, vii, viii, xi, xv, xviii, 4, 12, 29, 31, 32, 34, 41, 42, 44, 49, 53, 54, 56, 58, 60, 64, 66, 70, 72, 79, 96, 97, 102, 128, 162, 164 (*see also* Spontaneous drawings, Directed drawings)
Dream interpretations, 8, 44
Drives (*see* Instincts, Transformation)
Dulicai, Dianne, xxiii, 14, 105
Dynamically oriented (*see* Art Therapy, Naumberg, Margaret)
Dynamic Distortion, 80, 89, 102

E

Educational Psychology, 36
Educators, xxi, 165
Ego (*see also* Development)
autonomous function of, viii, xx, 18, 25, 42, 134, 161, 164
conflict-free sphere of, xvi, xx
enhancement of, 11, 12
strengths, xviii, xx, 9, 13, 26, 27
substructure of, 42
weaknesses, xviii, xx, 13, 27
Egocentrism, 31, 33, 35, 57, 58, 66, 77, 192, 193
Electroconvulsive therapy, 12
Emotional
disorder, 13, 16, 30, 36, 60, 128, 134, 136, 142, 163, 164 (*see also specific disorders*)
overexcitability, 37
states, xii, 36
status, 83
Emotional development (*see* Development)
English, Spurgeon, 14
Environment, 23, 25, 32, 34, 36, 42, 44, 49, 58, 66, 67, 71, 75, 77, 79, 119, 138, 155, 162
illustrations of, *Fig. 36D* 122, *Fig. 38A & B* 126
Epistomology, 193
Equilibration, 95, 193
Equilibrium, 26, 43, 59, 77, 140

Erikson, Erik, 15
Evaluation, 65, 164 (*see also* Case illustrations and studies)
Expression, 3, 4, 5 (*see also* Process)
External boundaries (*see* Boundaries)
Externalization, 12, 21, 78, 87, 103, 106, 137
illustration of, *Fig. 32A & B* 110

F

Family, 106, 119, 152, 163
art therapy evaluation of, 105, *Fig. 30A & B* 107 (*see also* Kwiatkowska, Hanna)
Fantasy, xxi, 11, 14, 22, 25, 26, 44, 45, 49, 51, 63, 65, 79, 91, 106, 118, 120, 150, 158, 163
illustration of, *Fig. 37B* 124
Father, 8, 14, 24, 71, 79, 102, 112, 120, 143
Fear, 14, 38, 45, 79, 91, 102
Female, 8, 51, 53, 80, 90, 93, 101, 103, 112, 113, 119 (*see also* Identification, Identity)
illustrations of, *Fig. 16C & D* 85
Figurative knowledge, 193
Figure-ground relationships, 45, *Fig. 3* 48
Figures (*see* Human figures)
Fine, B. D., xxi, 26, 148
Fink, Paul, J., vii-ix, xxiii, 3, 6, 8
Flavell, J. H., 31
Forisha, B. D., 58, 60
Form, 46, 66, 67, 70, 71, 86, 112, 150
Formal operational period, 31, 34, 35, 39, 59, 193
Free associations, 8, 11, 19
Freud, Anna, ix, xx, 15, 17, 18, 19, 20, 22, 23, 24, 25, 26, 27, 28, 30, 63, 65, 66, 71, 95, 97, 134, 162
Freud, Sigmund, vii, ix, xi, xii, xiii, 16, 17, 22, 23, 28, 32, 59, 65
Functional invariates, 194

G

Galin, D., 43
Gantt, Lynda, 7, 14
Gardner, Howard, 30, 56
Genetic
endowment, 38, 42
impairment, 38, 165
Genital, 113 (*see also* Development)

Goldman, Morris J., 36
Goodenough, F. L., 44
Graphic representations, xix, 22, 43, 46, 66, 72, 77, 78, 86, 88, 93, 94, 99, 101, 105, 106, 165 (*see also* Drawings)
Gratification, 19, 27, 28
Greenspan, Stanley I., viii, ix, xx, 21, 22, 24, 25, 27, 28, 36, 40, 41, 42, 43, 44, 59, 65, 75, 77, 96, 97, 104, 135, 136, 139, 140, 148, 150, 163, 164
Groundline (*see* Baseline)
Guilt, 9, 19

H

Haber, R. N., 58
Hammer, Emanuel F., 4, 45
Happiness, 78
Haptic, 78, 79
Hardiman, G. W., 53, 54, 60, 78, 97
Harms, Ernest, xvii, 4
Hartman, Heinz, xx
Hate, 8, 25, 42, 97
Hatterer, Lawrence J., 39
Hattwick, L. B. W., 79
Hays, Ronald E., xvi
Hierarchal developmental model of defense mechanisms, xv, 63, 128, *Table 1* 61-62
Holt, Robert R., 40, 41
Hoopes, Janet, xxiii
Horizon line, 78, 81, 90
 illustration of, *Fig. 16A* 84
Horowitz, Mardi, 136
Hospitalization
 effect of, 72
Hostility, 12
Human figures, xii, 44, 45, 46, 49, 53, 67, 75, 78, 86, 88, 89, 97, 98, 104, 109, 112, 113, 143, 158 (*see also* Stick figures)
 illustrations of, *Fig. 5* 50, *Fig. 6* 57, *Fig. 37A* 124
 static, 78, 112, 137, 163
 test (*see* Psychological tests)
Hysteria, 18, 26
Hysterical character, 148

I

Id, 17, 18, 20, 27, 28 (*see also* Psychosexual theory)

derivatives of, 18
Identification, 17, 19, 23, 24, 26, 63, 71, 77, 80, 86, 90, 91, 93, 97, 99, 100, 101, 103, 105, 106, 113, 119, 120, 127, 143, 145, 146, 158
 definition of, *Table 2* 131
 illustrations of, *Fig. 28A & B* 103, *Fig. 31A & B* 108, *Fig. 32A & B* 110, *Fig. 35C & D* 117, *Fig. 36C* 122, *Fig. 37A* 124, *Fig. 38C & D* 127, *Fig. 42C* 147
 with the aggressor, 21, 22, 80, 86, 97, 109, 112, 113, 119, 143
 definition of, *Table 2* 132
 illustrations of, *Fig. 32A & B* 110, *Fig. 35C & D* 117, *Fig. 36B* 121, *Fig. 42A* 146
Identity (*see also* Development)
 sexual, 90, 98
Imagery
 formation of, xi, 18, 32, 33, 35, 41, 49, 55, 56, 58, 59, 88
 visual, viii, 43, 55, 58, 59
Images, 103, 161 (*see also* Drawings)
 bland, 136
 body, 78, 90, 98, 141, *Fig. 42A* 146
 horrible, 136
 lurid, 136
 primitive, 58, 66, 70, 98, 150
 realistic, 102, 148
 self, 81, 89, 113, 120, 139, 143, *Fig. 41D* 145
 static, viii, 55, 152
 unbidden, 136
Imagination, 83 (*see also* Creative process)
Imaginational overexcitability, 37
Imitation, 23, 35, 63, 70, 71, 75, 89, 93, 112, 127, 130, 137, 139
 definition of, *Table 2* 130
 illustrations of, *Fig. 34A & B* 114, *Fig. 35A & B* 116, *Fig. 38C & D* 127
Impulses (*see also* Development)
 control of, 10
 gratification of, 18, 23, 136
Incorporation, 23, 93, 145
 definition of, *Table 2* 129
Individualistic, 78
Individuation, 11, 22, 42, 67 (*see also* Separation — Individualtion)
Infantile neuroses, 95 (*see also* Neuroses)
Inhelder, B., 35, 55
Inhibition, 21, 28, 38, 163
Inner screen, 43, 65, 120, 123, 150

Instincts, xxi, 22, 26, 42 (*see also* Development)
Instinctual, 86
  wishes, 87
Intellectual
  accomplishments, 94
  overexcitability, 37
Intellectualization, 12, 21, 24, 27, 63, 112, 130, 148
  definition of, *Table 2* 130
Intelligence, 72, 161, 189 (*see also* Cognitive development)
  quotient, 44
  tests (*see* Psychological tests)
Intensity, 20
Internal boundaries (*see* Boundaries)
Internalization, 21, 23, 60, 67, 77, 103
International Journal of Art Psychotherapy, 4, 7
Interpersonal relationships, 75, 135 (*see also* Relationships)
Intervention, 65, 128, 134, 135, 165
Introjection, 19, 22, 23, 27, 63, 97, 103
  definition of, *Table 2* 131
Involutional depression, 12
Irreversibility, 33, 95, 194
Isolation, 17, 18, 21, 44, 68, 103, 109, 112, 130, 136, 139, 142, 150, 158, 162
  definition of, *Table 2* 130
  illustrations of, *Fig. 10* 69, *Fig. 34A & B* 114, *Fig. 35A & B* 116, *Fig. 35E* 118, *Fig. 36D* 122, *Fig. 39* 138, *Fig. 40A & B* 141, *Fig. 41A, B & C* 144, *Fig. 42A* 146
  of affect, 16, 69, 77, 80, 81, 86, 88, 89, 90, 96, 98, 100, 101, 106, 109, 112, 113, 119, 123, 126, 148
  definition of, *Table 2* 130
  illustrations of, *Fig. 16A* 84, *Fig. 19* 90, *Fig. 21* 92, *Fig. 22* 94, *Fig. 25A & B* 99, *Fig. 27A & B* 101, *Fig. 31A & B* 108, *Fig. 34C* 115, *Fig. 36D* 122, *Fig. 37B* 124, *Fig. 38B* 126, *Fig. 43A & B* 148

J

Jacksonian principles, 37
Jealousy, 26
Jones, Don, 6

K

Kaplan, L., 40

Kaye-Huntingdon, Susan, xvi
Kellogg, Rhoda, 45, 46, 49, 51, 53, 67
Kestenberg, Judith S., 21
King, Saul, 4
Klee, Paul, 161
Koppitz, E. M., ix, 45
Kramer, Edith, xvii, 3, 6, 8, 9, 14
Kris, Ernst, 39
Kubie, Lawrence S., 39
Kwiatkowska, Hanna, 13

L

Language, 162 (*see also* Speech, Verbal)
Latency, 23, 24, 25, 26, 28, 51, 78, 94, 95, 98, 119, 152, 162
Latent (*see* Unconscious)
Lateralization, 43
Learning, 120
  theory of, xviii, 43
Left brain (*see* Lateralization)
Levick, Myra F., vii, viii, ix, xi, xii, 3, 4, 7, 10, 11, 12, 14, 45, 46, 58, 105
Levy, Bernard, 5
Lewis, M. M., 34
Lewis, Nolan C., 4, 5
Libido, 17 (*see also* Development)
Lidz, Theodore, 135
Logical reasoning, 23, 40, 44, 75 (*see also* Reasoning Development)
Lord, Gary, 171, 185
Love, 8, 19, 25, 42, 97
Lowenfeld, Viktor, 53, 54, 71, 78

M

Machover, Karen, 44, 45
Magic, 17, 65
Magical thinking, 23, 24, 112, 135
Mahler, Margaret S., 22, 23, 67
Maladaptive, xv, xviii, xxi, 16, 28, 35, 152, 165 (*see also* Behavior)
Male, 8, 24, 53, 80, 90, 93, 101, 103, 112, 119 (*see also* Identification, Identity)
Mandala, 46, *Fig. 4* 50
Manipulation, 77
Masculine (*see* Identification)
Mastery, 22, 23, 32, 33, 46, 49, 71, 145
Memory
  evocative, 40
Menninger, Karl, 6
Mental (*see also* Disorder)

dysfunction, 22 (*see also* Organicity)
representation, 86 (*see also* Drawings)
retardation, xix, 10 (*see also* Organicity)
status, xii
Metapsychological profile, 20
Methodology, 10-11 (*see also* Art Therapy)
Mirroring, 13, 162
Moore, B. E., xxi, 26, 148
Mother, 8, 24, 72, 79, 113, 120, 138, 143, 150
Motivation, 42
Movement, 8, 83, 105, 106, 113, 119, 139, 163
Music, 81, 83
Mythology, 91

N

Nagera, Humberto, 39
Naumberg, Margaret, xvii, 4, 5, 8, 9, 14, 157
Neale, J. M., 35
Neurophysiology, 43
Neuroses, 150 (*see also specific disorders*)
infantile, 19
moderate, xvii
obsessional, 12, 17, 148
Non-verbal, xi, 9, 12, 43, 45, 118
Normal populations, ix, xix, 19, 22, 34, 47, 60, 64, 128, 136
Noy, Pincus, ix, 41, 43, 44, 59, 60, 65, 120

O

Object, 67, 70, 75, 78, 79, 109, 119, 142
inanimate, 49, 78
permanence, 32
relations, xxi, 35, 42 (*see also* Development)
Obsessional (*see also* Behavior)
behavior, 13, 18
rituals, 18, 19
rumination, 16
Obsessive compulsive neuroses, 12
O'Dell, Scott, 45, 46, 49, 51
Odier, C., 40
Oedipal, 66, 71, 75, 76, 77, 79, 86
conflict, 17, 24, 25, 26, 63, 65, 77, 89, 90, 100, 120, 127, 136
pre-, 20, *Fig. 38A & B* 126
resolution of, 24, 41, 78, 93
stage, xviii, 22, 27, 97, 98, 109, 112, 125,

126, 136, 139, 148
illustrations of, *Fig. 18* 88, *Fig. 20* 91, *Fig. 21* 92
Omnipotence, 65
Ontogenetic, 38
Operation, 194
Operative, 194
Oral, xviii, 27, 59 (*see also* Development)
Organic
impairment, 72
learning disorder, 141
Organicity, xviii, 155
Organization, 35, 37, 40, 43, 44, 53, 54, 56, 60, 66, 71, 77, 90, 105, 119, 122, 148, 194
Osborne, Leslie, xix

P

Paivio, A., 58
Parents, 105, 106, 127, 145
Participation, 33, 194-195
Pavlovian, 36
Pearson product moment correlation (*see* Statistical analysis)
Peer
groups, 97, 152
relationships, 57, 96, 163
Perception, 55, 60, 77, 123, 135, 136, 165
illustration of, *Fig. 37C* 125
Personality development (*see* Development)
Phallic, 30, 58, 162 (*see also* Development)
Phobias, 16
Physical illness, 10, 13, 55, 71
Piagetian theory, viii, xv, xvii, xx, 28, 31, 40, 41, 53, 59, 60, 65, 75, 95
Piaget, Jean, vii, viii, ix, xi, xii, xiii, 27, 29-35, 40, 53, 54, 55, 57, 60, 65, 66, 71, 94, 95, 97
Pictorial stage, 49, 78, 79
illustrations of, *Fig. 7* 52, *Fig. 14* 76
Piechowski, M. M., 36, 37, 38, 39, 40
Pine, Fred, 23
Piotrowski Zygmundt A., xi-xiii
Play, xxi, 18, 56, 72
Pleasure principle, 19, 65 (*see also* Development)
Ploger, Benjamin, 5
Positive disintegration
theory of, 37
Post-Oedipal, 22, 23, 24, 75, 77, 89, 113 (*see*

also Development)
Pre-adolescent, 115, 120
  illustrations of, *Fig 34C & D* 115, *Fig. 36* 123
Pre-conscious, 79
Pre-genital (*see* Anal, Development, Oral, Pre-phallic)
Pre-operational period, 33, 34, 41, 59, 66, 75, 77, 87, 88, 97, 98, 112, 113, 135, 148, 163, 195
Pre-phallic, 148, 151 (*see also* Development)
  illustrations of, *Fig. 43A & B* 149, *Fig. 46A & B* 151
Primary process, ix, 21, 39, 40, 41, 43, 44, 55, 59
Primitive levels (*see also* Development)
  illustrations of, *Fig. 29* 104, *Fig. 41D* 145, *Fig. 42B* 146, *Fig. 45A & B* 153, *Fig. 46A, B & C* 155, *Fig. 48A, B & C* 160
Prisoners, 10, 13
Problem solving, 60, 66, 119
Process (*see also* Primary process, Secondary process)
  creative, 12, 36, 38 (*see also* Art, Expression, Graphic representation)
  developmental, 56
  maturational, 164
  mental, xi, 101, 112, 136
  therapeutic, xviii, 8, 9, 10, 13, 14, 15, 143, 148, 157, 165
Prognosis, 143
Projection, 17, 19, 22, 23, 26, 43, 63, 65, 66, 67, 70, 80, 81, 86, 103, 106, 112, 120, 123, 134, 137, 145, 150
  definition of, *Table 2* 129
  illustration of, *Fig. 9* 68, *Fig. 16B* 84, *Fig. 32A & B* 110, *Fig. 34A & B* 114, *Fig. 35A & B* 116
Projective technique, 4 (*see also* Psychological tests)
Psychiatrists, 6, 26, 188
Psychiatry, vii, ix, xvi
Psychic structure, 22 (*see also* Development)
Psychoanalysis, 15, 17, 35, 41, 128
Psychoanalysts, xvii, 95, 185
Psychoanalytic theory, xv, xvii, xx, 8, 14, 15, 17, 24, 28, 29, 39, 40, 42, 51, 59, 65, 75, 77, 79, 96, 134, 147, 163
Psychodiagnosis, 164, 165 (*see also* Diagnosis)
  illustration of, *Fig. 48A, B & C* 160

Psychological tests, xix, 83, 140, 155, 189
Psychologists, vii, xvii, 26, 38, 44, 83, 142, 185, 188
Psychology, ix, xvi, 15, 36, 43, 128
Psychomotor excitability, 37
Psychopathology, 35, 105 (*see also* Behavior, Maladaptive, *and specific mental disorders*)
Psychosexual development, vii, xx (*see also* Development)
Psychosis, xvii, 11, 16, 17, 58, 135, 150, 158 (*see also specific disorders*)
  illustration of, *Fig. 45A & B* 153
Psychotherapists, xvi, 6
Psychotherapy, 15
Puzzles, 140
  dexterity in, 140

Q

Qualitative differences, 54, 78
Quantitative differences, 54, 78, 112

R

Radials, 46
Rage, 24, 78, 137
Rainbows, 79, *Fig. 15A* 82
Rappaport, David, xxi, 24, 27, 28, 67
Rapprochement, 23
Rationalization, 24, 63, 77, 105, 123
  definition of, *Table 2* 130
  illustration of, *Fig. 37C* 125
  simple, 96, 104
Reaction formation, 17, 18, 20, 24, 25, 63, 77, 80, 81, 96, 98, 104, 105, 120, 146
  definition of, *Table 2* 132
  illustration of, *Fig. 16C & D* 85
Realism, 33, 77, 195
Realistic images, 100 (*see also* Images)
Reality, 77
  adaptation to, xx, xxi, 19, 21 (*see also* Adaptation)
  awareness of, 41, 43, 65, 150 (*see also* Development)
  principle, (*see* Secondary process)
Reasoning, 34, 95
Rectangles, 45
Regression, 11, 17, 21, 22, 24, 26, 63, 67, 69, 71, 72, 80, 81, 86, 93, 98, 99, 100, 101, 102, 105, 109, 112, 119, 120, 139,

142, 148, 164
definition of, *Table 2* 132
illustrations of, *Fig 9* 68, *Fig. 12A* 73, *Fig. 16C & D* 85, *Fig. 17* 87, *Fig. 24A & B* 96, *Fig. 25A & B* 99, *Fig. 27A & B* 101, *Fig. 30A & B* 107, *Fig. 33 A & B* 111, *Fig. 34D* 115, *Fig. 35A & B* 116, *Fig. 35E* 118, *Fig. 36A* 121, *Fig. 40A & B* 141, *Fig. 41A, B & C* 144, *Fig. 42A* 146, *Fig. 45A & B* 153
Relationships, 79, 81
  dyadic, 77, 89
  pictorial objects, between, 93, 97, 109
  spacial, 54, 90, 105, 119, 150
  therapeutic, 3, 13
  transference, 8, 9
  triangular, 41, 75, 77, 89
Reliability, xvi
  study of, 64, 171-183, *Tables 3-6* 172-182
Representational, xxi, 40, 41, 42, 54, 56, 65, 70, 78
Repression, xxi, 17, 18, 20, 21, 23, 25, 26, 63, 96, 100, 101, 119, 125, 136, 158, 163
definition of, *Table 2* 132
illustrations of, *Fig. 28A & B* 103, *Fig. 36C* 122, *Fig. 37B* 124
Resistance, xxi, (*see also* Adaptation, Defenses)
Reversability, 20, 25, 195
Reversal, 19, 21, 43, 63, 80, 81, 97, 98, 105, 120, 123, 142, 143, 150
definition of, *Table 2* 131
illustrations of, *Fig. 16C & D* 85, *Fig. 30A & B* 107, *Fig. 37A* 124, *Fig. 41A, B & C* 144
Rhythm, 8
Right brain (*see* Lateralization)
Role identification (*see* Identification, Development)
Role taking, 195
Rosen, Hugh, viii, 30, 31, 32, 33, 35, 57, 58, 65, 95, 135, 136
Rorschach (*see* Psychological tests)
Rothgeb, C. L., 16, 23, 65

S

Schema, xvi, 53, 54, 70, 71, 112, 125, 165
Schematic, 43 (*see also* Artistic development)
Scheme, 195
Schizophrenia, 135, 136, 150, 157 (*see also* Case illustrations and studies)
  chronic, xii, 11, 152, *Fig. 47A, B & C* 157
  paranoid, 11, 152, *Fig. 46A, B & C* 155
Scribbles, 45, 56, 63, 65, 66, 67, 70, 71, 80, 86, 93, 100, 112, 119, 161, *Fig. 1A & B* 47
Secondary elaboration, 8 (*see also* Secondary process)
Secondary process, viii, 24, 39, 40, 43, 44, 59, 99
Self (*see also* Images)
  images of, *Fig. 26A & B* 100
Semiotic function, 32, 195
Sensorimotor period, 31, 59, 195
Sensual overexcitability, 37
Separation, 11, 22, 42, 135
  and individuation, 67, 140, 148
Sequence (*see* Development)
Seriation, 34
Sexual, 163 (*see also* Instincts, Transformation)
  abuse, 127
Shapes within shapes, 45, 46, 49, 66, 71, 102, 113, 119
  illustrations of, *Fig. 2A & B* 148, *Fig. 36A* 121, *Fig. 36D* 122
Siblings, 24, 80, 119, 120, 126, 141, 142
Signifier, 196
Signs, 32, 33, 55, 81
Snyder, Sam, xxiii, 45
Sociocentric, 196
Space, 8, 32, 71
Spatial relationships (*see* Relationships)
Speech
  egocentric, 57, 60
  socialized, 57
  symbolic, 4, 5, 57
Splitting, 145 (*see also* Isolation of affect)
Spontaneous Drawings, vii, xv, xvi, xvii, xx, 5, 11, 14, 18, 42, 46, 75, 79, 102, 103, 119, 135, 147, 164, 188
Squares, 45, 46, 95
Stability, 18, 27, 150
Stages (*see* Developmental, *and specific stages*
Statistical analysis (*see* Reliability, Validity)
Stern, Max, 4
Stick figures, 49, 86, 93, 98, 100, 163 (*see also* Human figure)
Stimuli, 40
Straus, M., 7, 14

Stress, 105, 106, 135
Structural (*see* Piagetian theory)
Structures (*see* Piaget)
Styles of drawing, 101 (*see also* Drawings)
Sublimation, 17, 63, 80, 86, 87, 89, 91, 105, 109
Substitute formation, 79
Sun, 46, 49, 75, 90, 112
Superego, 17, 18, 19, 24, 27, 28, 96 (*see also* Development)
Surrogate, 55, 79
Symbiotic (*see also* Relationships)
  patterns, 41
  relationships, 139, 140, 152
Symbolic
  process, viii, 8, 33, 78, 80, 87, 88, 104, *Fig. 20* 91
  representation, 101, 102, 112, 148, 150, 161, *Fig. 37C* 125
Symbolism, 53, 65, 89, 136, *Fig. 38A* 126
  definition of, *Table 2* 129
Symbols, 32, 33, 35, 41, 55, 56, 70, 71, 75, 81, 87, 90, 98, *Fig. 14* 76

T

Theory (*see* specific theory)
Therapeutic process (*see* Process)
Training (*see* Art Therapy)
Transduction, 196
Transference, 148
Transformations, 18, 25, 33, 36, 37, 40, 54, 89, 119, 123, 136, 150
  illustrations of, *Fig. 36D* 122
Transitional, *Fig. 36A* 121 (*see also* Development sequences)
Trauma, *Fig. 48A, B & C* 160 (*see also* Case illustrations and studies)

Triangles, 45
Turning against the self, 19, 21

U

Ulman, Elinor, xvii, 5, 6, 7, 8, 9
Unbidden images (*see* Images)
Unconscious, 8, 13, 18, 26, 42, 89, 97
  wishes, 79
Undoing, 17, 63, 72, 75, 93, 98, 99, 102, 105, 106, 112, 113, 119, 120, 142, 143, 148
  definition of, *Table 2* 131
  illustration of, *Fig. 24A & B* 96, *Fig. 25A & B* 99, *Fig. 29* 104, *Fig. 30A & B* 107, *Fig. 34C & D* 115, *Fig. 36A* 121, *Fig. 41A, B & C* 144, *Fig. 42A* 146, *Fig. 43A & B* 149

V

Vaccaro, V. Michael, xxiii, 14
Validity
  study of, 184-189, *Tables 7-11* 184-189
Verbal, 72, 123, 150, 163
Vygotsky, Lev S., 57, 58

W

Wallace, Edith, 7
Wechsler Object Assembly Test (*see* Psychological tests)
Withdrawal, 69, 158, 162
Wolff, Peter H., 36, 40

Z

Zernick, T., 53, 78, 97
Zetzel, E., 25, 28, 54, 60
Zwerling, Israel, xxiii, 15